Contents

Introduction

The World Health Organisation estimates that about 14 million people are currently infected with the human immunodeficiency virus worldwide. Of these, over one million are women, and one half of all newly-infected people are women. By the year 2000, 13 million women may be infected with the virus, and consequently, between one-fifth and one-third of their children too.

An epidemic which was initially labelled as being a 'gay plague', is now spreading most rapidly by the heterosexual route. Half of the infected people are in the group defined by the World Health Organisation as 'young people', the 15-24 years age group. This is the group which in many societies is bearing the greatest burden of social responsibility, of work and childrearing. Women are now facing the full force of the infection globally, by becoming infected and widowed, having to take on the role of family provider as well as carer. Subsequently, children also become affected and infected, adding to the emotional strain of their mothers.

Women are susceptible to HIV infection in many ways. Women are socially vulnerable in most areas of the world. It is common for double standards of fidelity to exist, with monogamy expected of the woman, and multiple partners accepted for men. There is often sexual subordination, with women retaining little choice or control in sexual matters, finding it difficult to protect themselves when they may fear or know they may be at risk. Physiologically they have a large mucosal area of exposure to infected semen, which itself contains higher concentrations of virus than vaginal secretions. Increasingly, men are seeking out virgins in the expectation that they will be safe from infection. The rupture of the hymen, and the younger age at which a man may be certain of achieving this aim, renders the young girl susceptible to infection from tissue damage. Women are frequently economically dependent, in some situations politically and legally impotent, and educationally repressed. Dr Merson of the WHO cited these points at a Conference held specifically to discuss the issues of HIV relating to women and children. This was only the second such conference to be held, when others have become an annual event.

HIV Infection in Pregnancy

Caroline M. Shepherd
RN, RM, ADM, PGCEA

Books for Midwives Press
Books for Midwives Press is a joint publishing venture
between The Royal College of Midwives and
Haigh & Hochland Publications Ltd

Published by Books for Midwives Press, 174a Ashley Road, Hale, Cheshire, WA15 9SF, England

© 1994, Caroline M. Shepherd First edition

ISBN 1-898507-06-6

British Library Cataloguing in Publication Data
A catalogue record for this book is available from the British Library

Printed in Great Britain by RAP Ltd

Acknowledgements

I would firstly like to thank Betty Sweet, who introduced me to the possibility of writing a book. She has followed up this grave responsibility up by continued help and advice throughout, and her promptly returned pertinent comments have given me so much encouragement.

I would like to express my appreciation to Sue Cammerloher, retired midwife teacher, whose inimitable style and professionalism have always inspired me, and without whom I may never have become involved with HIV. Sue has made an enormous contribution to the care of women by her careful, thoughtful and thorough preparation of their carers, enabling and encouraging midwives to practice safely and compassionately.

I owe a debt of gratitude to Dr Alan Tang, Consultant in Genito-Urinary Medicine, who has given me so much of his time and help in the preparation of this book. He has willingly acted as a resource for my search for information, and as a constructive critic of the results.

Lastly, my thanks to Henry Hochland, who has never ceased to give me encouragement, and always without hassle, two very necessary ingredients in the production of a book.

The issues of HIV infection relating to women and their children are manifold and affect one of the most powerful human instincts and needs: that of procreating life. HIV and AIDS has been linked to 'sexual impropriety' from the outset. This has made the subject a taboo and has caused pain, misery and solitude for all who have fallen under its shadow. It has prevented people from coming forward for testing and treatment, and this association has led to a false sense of security for those not belonging to the so-called 'risk groups'.

Knowledge about the virus, its action and effect on the immune system is continually developing, changing the management of the disease and the direction of the research. Information and advice continues to be provisional, the goalposts changing as new discoveries surpass the previous. For the woman there are choices to be made: about being tested, what are the benefits? Should she have a child? What are the risks? To her baby, to her? These questions will have different answers depending upon where she happens to live. Resources vary dramatically from continent to continent, country to country, and even within communities. Social deprivation and HIV disease impact upon each other, compounding and causing problems in equal measure, like two strands of DNA. It is useful to examine the different elements in order to understand the whole.

CHAPTER 1

The Virus

The Human Immunodeficiency Virus(HIV) was identified by Luc Montagnier as the causative organism of the Acquired Immunodeficiency Syndrome (AIDS) in 1984, in France. Researchers from both sides of the Atlantic came to the discovery at much the same time, but called the virus by different names: the lymphadenopathy associated virus (LAV), Human T-cell leukaemia (lymphadenopathy) virus type III (HTLV-III), and AIDS-associated retrovirus (ARV). In 1986 it was decided to designate the AIDS retroviruses as 'human immuno-deficiency viruses'.

Structure of the virus

Viruses are composed of a core of nucleic acid, constituting the viral genome, and a protective outer shell made of protein or lipoprotein. The proteins in this shell, or capsid, have an affinity for receptor sites on host cells, which allows the virus to enter the cell in order to reproduce, as a virus is unable to reproduce outside of a host cell. The nucleic acid consists either of deoxyribonucleic acid (DNA), or ribonucleic acid (RNA), allowing the cell to reproduce. HIV is a *retrovirus*, an RNA virus characterized by having a viral enzyme, *reverse transcriptase,* which allows the virus to make a DNA copy of its RNA genetic material. The proteins on the shell have been identified and labelled (Figure 1.1) .

How the Virus Acts

1. The outer proteins act as antigenic 'keys' which have an affinity for receptor sites or 'locks' on the host cell. The receptor site for HIV has been labelled the CD4 receptor. Once attached the virus is able to gain entry through the cell membrane, and release its contents into the host cell. It was hoped that it may be possible to inhibit the binding of HIV to the CD4 receptor by either using antibodies to the gp120 and gp41 proteins or by using soluble CD4 to block receptor sites. Neither of these solutions has been successful to date.

Figure 1.1: Structure of HIV cell

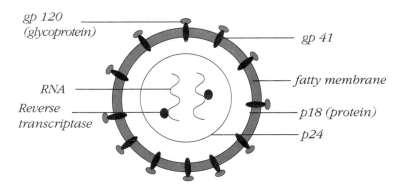

gp 120 (glycoprotein)

gp 41

RNA

fatty membrane

Reverse transcriptase

p18 (protein)

p24

2. The reverse transcriptase enables the viral genome to copy itself from RNA to DNA genetic material, and enter the nucleus of the host cell, becoming incorporated into the DNA of the host cell, making the virus a permanent part of the cell. This action is often referred to as 'piracy'. Much research has centred on blocking the action of reverse transcriptase, thus preventing the virus from becoming incorporated into the cell.

3. Once incorporated into the host cell, the virus can replicate itself whenever the cell would be stimulated to reproduce itself. There are specific genes that are responsible for activity and replication, and research is being done into interrupting the cycle at these points: by inhibiting those genes responsible for increasing HIV activity, and the production of viral RNA and proteins.

4. As the virus production within the cell increases, the cell membrane ruptures, releasing the new viruses, a process known as 'budding'. The viruses surround themselves with their lipoprotein coat, collected from cytoplasm of the host cell membrane. Scientists are also hoping to develop an inhibitor to the enzyme which assembles the enzymes and proteins necessary for the maturation of the virus prior to budding.

5. The new virus cells circulate in the bloodstream seeking new cells with CD4 receptors. The host cell is perforated by the budding process, the contents leak out, and cell death follows.

6.   CD4 receptors on the T4 lymphocytes and the viral antigens have a high affinity for each other. This results in many uninfected cells binding to the infected cell and merging with it, forming large bodies called syncitia. A syncitium cannot function and subsequently dies. Thus although only one T4 cell may have been infected, hundreds of other non-infected cells may die with it. (Redfield and Burke, 1988)

As a response to infection by the virus, the immune system will manufacture antibodies. These antibodiesare non-neutralizing, and do not afford protection from further infection. It usually takes three months for these antibodies to be present, during which time the individual is infectious, but will test negative to HIV antibody testing. This antibody-free period is known as the 'window period'.

EFFECTS OF THE HIV ON THE BODY

An Overview Of The Immune System

The immune system is comprised of specific and non-specific mechanisms of protection from infectious disease.

Non-specific immunity consists of the following.
*   Prevention of infection, primarily by intact skin; each orifice or break in this protection is itself protected by a range of measures, such as ciliated cells and mucous membranes, pH changes, and chemical secretions (e.g. lysozymes in tears).

*   Containment of infection, (a) by the process of inflammation - the area of invasion has an increased blood supply bringing protective cells and phagocytes, and, (b) by phagocytosis, where bacteria are engulfed and destroyed by white cells, including macrophages.

This often leads to a successful conclusion of the infection.

Specific immunity is acquired to afford protection from organisms which are more hostile or overwhelming. It may be divided into two types: *humoral,* and *cell-mediated* immunity, both involving lymphocytes.

Humoral immunity concerns B-lymphocytes, which like T-lymphocytes originate from stem cells in the bone marrow.

B-lymphocytes amount to 30 per cent of the total number of lymphocytes and act on specific antigens. In response to infection B-cells proliferate and change into plasma cells, secreting antibody to combine with the antigen and incapacitate it, eventually destroying it by a process of lysis. Memory cells are also formed, to enable a rapid response to future infection by the same antigen.

Figure 1.2: Diagram to illustrate specific immunity

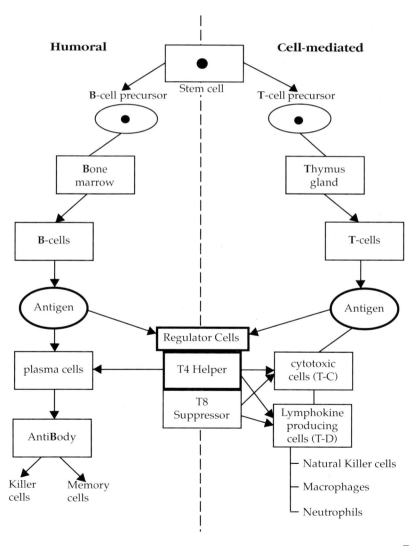

Cell-mediated immunity concerns T-lymphocytes which account for 70 per cent of lymphocytes and have differing functions. T-D cells (lymphokines), produce substances which interact with other inflammatory and phagocytic cells substances and destroy cells. Some lymphokines, such as interferon, have a direct antivirus effect, and can also activate cells known as Natural Killer or NK cells. These cells target pre-tumorous cells and protect the body from neoplastic disease. T-C cells, when activated by T-helper cells, are able to destroy cells which contain virus, and are known as cytotoxic cells (Pratt, 1991).

All lymphocytes are regulated by two types of cells: *helper* cells, which are also known as T4 lymphocytes, initiate both the B- and T-lymphocyte activity (i.e. the secretion of specific antibody by the plasma cells), and the cytotoxic and lymphokine-producing T-lymphocytes; and *suppressor* cells, known as T8 cells, which suppress the helper, cytotoxic and lymphokine-producing cells when the need is over. The normal ratio of T4: T8 cells is 2:1.

Effects Of HIV On The Immune System

The HIV receptor sites are present in different types of cells within the body. This particular receptor on the host cell has become known as the CD4 marker, and has been found on a variety of cells, most notably T4 lymphocytes but also on some macrophages and certain glial cells within the central nervous system. Cells containing the CD4 marker have become known generically as CD4 cells.

Once HIV has entered the T4 cell, it remains there until the cell is stimulated to reproduce. Once this helper cell is activated it will produce virus, and will itself be destroyed. It will be activated by the presence of infections or by the presence of non-infective antigens, such as are found in semen. The newly-produced viruses bud out from the cells, killing the host helper cell, and infect other helper cells. It is also thought that cells containing HIV may exert an auto-immune response against non-infected T4 cells, resulting in a further destruction of these cells.

The functions of the T4 helper cells are interfered with by a reduction in their number.

- B lymphocytes need T4 lymphocytes to help them to produce specific antibodies to specific antigens. Immunity from specific infection is acquired throughout life both actively and passively. Many infections do not become evident, because antibodies are released at the first signal of invasion, and the infection is contained. Should these specific antibodies not be stimulated, infections 'take their opportunity' to invade, and infections to which the body was previously immune are allowed to resurface. Such opportunistic infections include herpes, cytomegalovirus and candida.

• Lymphokine and cytotoxic cell production is impaired which results in neoplastic and viral cells not being destroyed. One of the diseases associated with AIDS is Kaposi's Sarcoma, a neoplastic disease.

• The T4 helper: T8 suppressor ratio is disturbed, resulting in a lowered response to infection.

Transmission of the virus

The virus is primarily blood borne, although it has been isolated in other body fluids, namely semen, vaginal secretions, breast-milk, tears, saliva and cerebrospinal fluid. The routes of transmission are:

Vertical   —   transplacental and perinatal;

Horizontal —   sexual activity, where there is exchange
                 of or contact with body fluids;
            —   transfusion:
                 —   infected blood through sharing needles in
                      intravenous drug misuse;
                 —   infected blood or blood products from
                      donor;
            —   organ transplantation or artificial insemination
                 by donor semen.

Historically, sexual intercourse has been the primary route of HIV transmission. In the western world the epidemic began mainly among the gay population, with homosexual men accounting for the largest group of individuals with the disease. Factors facilitating transmission include lesions or broken skin, thus the coexistence of other sexually transmitted diseases such as syphilis or genital herpes, and sexual practices such as anal intercourse which may damage the rectal mucosa, are likely to increase the efficiency of transmission.

In Africa, the spread of HIV has always been associated with heterosexual activity. The depositing of infected semen, at a velocity of approximately ten miles per hour, within the vagina renders the woman more susceptible to infection than the man may be from infected vaginal and cervical secretions. The infectivity rate of man to woman is thought to be approximately a 22 per cent chance with each sexual act, whereas, it is nine per cent from woman to man (Padian *et al*, 1990).

Heterosexual activity has become the principal mode of transmission worldwide. It follows that vertical transmission, i.e. from mother to child, will become of increasing significance. The mother-to-child transmission rate has been studied worldwide with differing rates being discovered in different continents. Various studies had used differing methods and criteria for assessing transmission, and since 1992 there has been a consensus arrived at in the reporting of figures. This has allowed comparison of the figures, and has confirmed what has been evident for years, that there is a disparity in transmission rates between the developed and the developing countries. Transmission rates in non-industrialized countries are virtually double those in industrialized countries. The reason for this is not clearly understood, but may be associated with the general health of the women in these countries, and with the presence of malaria and other intercurrent infections.

HIV, having been cultured from eight week fetuses, must be able to cross the placental barrier. The mechanism of infection is not clearly known, but may well involve invasion by HIV of the syncitial layer and of the trophoblast itself. What is also not known is why some fetuses are infected and why some are not. Currently it is not possible either to predict which pregnancies may be affected, or to prevent transmission. It appears that the combined rate of transmission occurring at delivery and postnatally is higher than transplacental transmission. From studies mainly in Africa, it appears that the risk of transmission antenatally is 35 per cent, intrapartum figures are 18 per cent, and postnatal infection, comprised almost exclusively from breastfeeding, is between 14 and 26 per cent (Van de Perre, 1993; Dunn *et al*, 1993).

Transmission from infected donor blood, blood products and organs is now a much lower risk, as all donated products are tested for HIV antibodies. Potential donors from known high risk groups are also asked to exclude themselves. Although substantially reducing the risk, the existence of the window period in those persons who do not belong to the known high risk groups, but whom may be infected does not eliminate infection through this route.

Intravenous drug users sharing infected needles and syringes account for a major proportion of HIV infection. 'Sharing works' forms part of the drug-using culture in some areas, and sexual activity spreads the disease into the wider population. The need for money to buy the drugs necessary for the addiction forces many users into prostitution, and sex without a condom may bring in more money. The introduction of needle exchanges and prescribed drugs has made the addiction to these substances more controlled and less hazardous. A regular supply of drugs and equipment has reduced the need for prostitution to buy the drugs, and for sharing needles and syringes.

Knowledge of the routes of transmission led to the terminology of 'at risk groups', meaning groups of people who were at risk of contracting the disease through their behaviour. Included in this were homosexual and bisexual men, intravenous drug users, people from sub-Saharan Africa. This has resulted in individuals being discriminated against for their membership of a group rather than their behaviour. The term 'at risk behaviour' denotes the risky activity rather than the individual, who although belonging to a particular group deemed to be at risk, may not be participating in at risk behaviour.

CHAPTER 2

Epidemiology

In the early years of the AIDS epidemic, the spread of the disease was understood to be through the homosexual community, mainly in New York and San Francisco. Increasing numbers of deaths were occurring among formerly fit young men. The name initially given to the syndrome of unexplained immune deficiency was GRID - Gay Related Immune Deficiency. The next group of people noted to display the same curious symptoms were intravenous drug users, closely followed in Miami by immigrants from Haiti. For the first time, women were found to be among the immigrants suffering from this disease. Once the cause of the disease was confirmed to be a virus, much debate ensued about where the virus originated, and why these three 'H' groups (Homosexual, Heroin and Haiti) came to be simultaneously infected. The origin of the virus has never been established and in current times ceases to be of importance. Much more relevant is the monitoring of how the disease is spreading currently.

Throughout the 1980s AIDS became prevalent throughout the world. Almost from the start there were widely varying patterns of spread. In North America, Latin America, Oceania and Western Europe the cases of AIDS were predominantly among young and middle-aged gay men, with very small numbers of women and children affected. In sub-Saharan Africa, the picture was different, with more than half the number of infections occurring in women and children.

The World Health Organisation (WHO) described the spread in terms of epidemiological patterns according to dominant mode of transmission (Chin and Mann, 1988).

Worldwide it is estimated that one-third of all those infected by HIV are women. The WHO predicts that by the year 2000, the figures will be almost equal between men and women. Figure 2.1 shows the WHO estimation of the infection rates among women.

Table 2.1: The World Health Organisation's classification of the spread of HIV

	Areas	**Mode of Transmission**	**Began**
Pattern I	North America, Oceania, Western Europe	Homosexuals, intravenous drug users	Late 1970's, early 1980's
Pattern II	Sub-Saharan Africa, Caribbean	Heterosexual, Perinatal becoming of increasing significance	Late 1970's
Pattern I/II	Latin America	Initially homosexual, becoming heterosexual	1980's
Pattern III	Asia, Pacific (excluding Australia and New Zealand), Eastern Europe, North Africa, Middle East	Initially no clear route, latterly intravenous drug use, and prostitution	1980's

Figure 2.1: Estimated number of HIV-1 infected women aged 15-49 years. No. in boxes = prevalence per 100,000 women (Source: World Health Organisation, 1991)

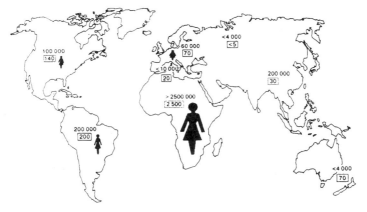

By 1990 there were more than three million women infected with HIV, most of them were of child-bearing age and about 80 per cent lived in sub-Saharan Africa. Although the dominant mode of transmission is heterosexual intercourse, it is estimated that ten per cent of women have become infected through a blood transfusion. The facilities for HIV testing may not be readily available in these countries, and the many pregnancies these women have and their often poor physical health renders them more likely to have to receive a blood transfusion.

At present 3,000 women become infected, and 500 women die each day from an AIDS-related illness. Most of these are in the 15-24 year age group. Of all newly infected people, 50 per cent are women. The WHO estimates that by the year 2000, 13 million women will have been infected (Merson, 1993). Given that the mother-to-child transmission rate in Africa is 30 per cent, this means that one-third of the children of these women will also become infected. Children will become victims of the disease, by either developing the disease, by being orphaned, or both.

In nine American cities AIDS is the commonest cause of death and in southern Africa infected women now outnumber men 6:5, and up to 35-40 per cent of women attending antenatal clinics in sub-Saharan Africa are known to be HIV positive (Merson, 1993).

In the United Kingdom, at the end of 1991, only five per cent of people with AIDS were women. The period between becoming infected with HIV and developing AIDS is on average 8-10 years. Figures for people with AIDS reflect infection that took place ten years ago. The figures for people with HIV infection inform us of the current infection, and of future AIDS predictions. Women with HIV infection and AIDS account for 12 per cent of those infected. Gay men and haemophiliacs with HIV infection is reducing in proportion to those with AIDS, whilst those infected with HIV through intravenous drug use and heterosexual activity is rising. This demonstrates a significant shift in mode of transmission.

In the AIDS and HIV-1 infection in the United Kingdom report for January 1994 it is noted that in the two years 1992 and 1993, the number of AIDS cases reported rose overall by nine per cent.

Exposure through heterosexual intercourse accounted for 13 per cent of the cumulative figures (from 1982-1992). The 1994 report states that 30 per cent of AIDS cases, and 38 per cent of HIV-1 infection reported in 1993 was attributed to heterosexual men and women.

Table 2.2: Illustration of the increase in AIDS cases in women over two years

	1992	**1993**	**Increase**
Male AIDS cases	1,341	1,404	5%
Female AIDS cases	142	215	51% (18% in 1992)

CHAPTER 3

The HIV-AIDS Spectrum

Seroconversion

Seroconversion to an HIV-Positive state may occur at any time from a few days to three months post-infection. It has been reported that at the time of seroconversion there may be a short flu-like illness, but this appears to occur in the minority of people. As many people are unaware that they have been infected, this viral-type illness may be put down to one of the many acute, but short-lived viral infections that circulate within the population. After seroconversion occurs the individual may remain well and symptom-free for a considerable period of time.

Progression from HIV to AIDS

It is currently thought that everyone with HIV infection will remain so and infectious for life. It is not yet known if all of them will become ill, or will die as a result. Most of them will probably de- velop some ill-health as a result of the compromise of their immune system. WHO studies indicate that there is not much difference in the progression rate to AIDS between areas or modes of transmis- sion. Their data shows that 20 per cent of infected individuals will progress to AIDS in five years, and 50 per cent of people within ten years. There are no data available beyond ten years, but the predic- tion is that progression may be 75 per cent within 15 years, and 95 per cent in 20 years (Chin, 1990). As it is often difficult for an indi- vidual to assess when they were infected, it is not easy to gain an accurate picture of the disease process. The WHO use serological data and epidemiological observations of when HIV infection first spread into the population. Most of the data comes from studies of HIV infection in gay men (Rutherford *et al*, 1990), and it is to be noted that similar long-term studies of HIV infection among drug users or women have not been completed.

The progression to AIDS is fairly constant in the adult disease, but paediatric AIDS progression is much swifter, with an estimated 17 per cent of deaths occurring within the first year of life. The WHO model of progression to paediatric AIDS status is 25 per cent within the first year, 45 per cent in the second, 60 per cent in the third, and 80 per cent in the fourth.

Signs and Symptoms

The first symptom of HIV disease is often enlarged lymph nodes. This may last for several years and not be associated with any other form of disease. Other symptoms which begin to occur are weight loss, fevers, night sweats, diarrhoea and oral candidiasis. Both men and women are prone to oral thrush, and candidiasis may occur throughout the digestive tract, causing immense discomfort. Women commonly develop vaginal thrush which recurs and is very hard to treat successfully. Women are also very prone to other gynaecological infections such as genital warts, genital herpes, and pelvic inflammatory disease. These may be recurrent and severe. In addition when the immune system becomes compromised, the usual indicators of infection such as pain and inflammation may not be present, masking the infection and delaying diagnosis and treatment. There is evidence that women are more likely to develop abnormal cervical smears, with some progressing to cervical cancer.

Laboratory tests may demonstrate a reduction in T4 cell count, a reduction in the T4:T8 ratio, leucopenia, lymphopenia, and raised levels of immunoglobulin.

These signs and symptoms were collectively named as ARC - AIDS Related Complex, although this term is not currently used much. As the immune system becomes more compromised by the virus, opportunistic infections may occur. These are infections that the immune system commonly keeps suppressed by the use of cell-mediated immunity, i.e. the memory cells initiate the production of specific antibodies, triggered by the T4 lymphocyte. As the T4 cell count falls this immunity is suppressed and infection results. Examples of such infections are herpes simplex, cytomegalovirus and toxoplasmosis.

Major opportunistic infections such as pneumocystis carinii pneumonia (PCP) are diagnostic of AIDS. Cancers such as Kaposi's Sarcoma (KS) are also indicative of AIDS. Kaposi's Sarcoma is a less common manifestation in women, and is seldom seen among women who have contracted the disease through needle-sharing. Women who have contracted HIV infection through sex are more likely to develop KS if their partner was bisexual. If women do develop KS it may spread more rapidly than in men, and often proves fatal. (Lassoued *et al*, 1991).

Classification of AIDS

The Centre for Disease Control (CDC) developed a classification system for HIV infection and AIDS in 1986 and 1987, upon which many medical treatment and social welfare programmes were based. This classification listed all the clinical conditions and laboratory markers that would define whether an individual would be given an AIDS diagnosis. With further knowledge about the pattern of the disease, and the significance of such predictive markers as the CD4 cell count, the CDC issued a new classification in December 1992. An AIDS diagnosis now includes all HIV-infected persons with <200 CD4+ T-lymphocytes/microlitre, or a CD4+ T-lymphocytes percentage of total lymphocytes of <14. This will have the potential of dramatically increasing the numbers of people with an AIDS diagnosis, as many people will have a CD4 cell count of <200, but no clinical symptoms, on which the previous classification was based. Chaisson *et al* (1993) estimated that it would double the number of cases. This has important implications for the medical and social services provision, as many programmes including disability benefits, and support networks rely on an AIDS diagnosis for entitlement.

The 1993 Classification also added three medical conditions to the diagnosis of AIDS (see Appendix I). These are pulmonary tuberculosis, recurrent pneumonia and invasive cervical cancer. This will lead to more women and drug users meeting the criteria. Women have often been under-represented in AIDS figures, as gynaecological conditions were not included. This reduced their entitlement to benefits and also inclusion in drug trials which are sometimes dependent on an AIDS diagnosis for recruitment. However, Chaisson *et al* (1993) comment that, "while cervical dysplasia intraepithelial and squamous intraepithelial lesions are common in HIV-infected women, especially those with low CD4 counts, invasive cancer appears to be rare".

CHAPTER 4

The Effect of HIV on Pregnancy

As with many other areas concerning HIV infection, the effects that HIV has on a pregnancy are not well understood. Concerns have been raised about the physiological facts of transmission of the virus to the fetus, teratogenic effects of the virus on the developing fetus, increased pregnancy loss, decision to terminate the pregnancy, effects of drug therapy, and obstetric interventions. These areas have been studied, but many studies have been subject to the limitations of the relatively small number of diagnosed HIV positive women. Equally important but less measurable are the psychological effects of the disease which will also be discussed in a later chapter.

Perinatal transmission

It is known that the virus can cross the placental barrier, and will infect some fetuses. Babies of HIV positive mothers will carry the HIV antibodies formed by their mothers. It may take up to 18 months for these antibodies to be shed, an immensely long period of worry. It is now possible, however, to gain an earlier diagnosis with the availability of direct antigen tests. These tests are able to detect the presence of the HIV proteins (or antigens) and nucleic acids, indicating presence of the virus.

Initially, estimates of mother-to-child transmission of the virus were as high as 65 per cent per pregnancy. These early figures were gained from retrospective case studies, and may have been skewed by the small numbers involved and by the advanced disease progression of the women studied. In order to gain a more accurate picture of the effects of the virus on pregnancy and infants, a prospective collaborative study was set up Europe-wide. It was necessary to pool information as the numbers of known infected women per country were still relatively small. Many of the infected women were intravenous drug-users, or partners of drug-users, which may have a bearing on the data as the effects of substance abuse on the fetus needed to be assessed in addition to the effect of HIV.

Many other countries worldwide had also studied the perinatal transmission rate, and most had used differing methods to collect their data. In 1992 an international group of researchers met in Ghent, Belgium to estimate the mother-to-child transmission rate and to co-ordinate all the work being carried out. By then, there had been 14 studies published which had all used different methods to calculate the rate. Broadly, and taken as a whole, they reported a transmission rate of 12-30 per cent in industrialized countries, and 25-49 per cent in non-industrialized countries. They agreed upon a method of reporting data, ensuring that there was standardization of criteria and types of tests used. The Ghent researchers in 1992 thus achieved a way of utilizing data concordantly, and thereby achieving an overall mother-to-child transmission rate. Using this method, the Ghent researchers in 1993 reported that the European Collaborative Study transmission rate was 16.6%±1.5%. Sub-Saharan rates were 28 per cent ± 2.5 per cent.

It has been estimated that only 35 per cent of transmission will occur antenatally, with 65 per cent occurring either at delivery or postpartum (Temmerman, 1993). The biological mechanisms of transmission are not understood. The hypotheses include trophoblastic invasion by HIV, placental inflammation, the immune-suppression of pregnancy causing ascending infection of the genital tract and a resulting chorio-amnionitis, and the disease stage of the mother. However, mother-to-child transmission does not appear to be associated with parity, drug use, race or age of the mother (Newell, 1993). It appears that a mother who has recently become infected, or who is demonstrating signs of disease progression, i.e. becoming symptomatic and whose CD4 count is falling, may transmit the virus more effectively. It is also hypothesized that different strains of HIV-1 may transmit more effectively (Hague *et al*, 1993). One study in Canada has suggested that previous miscarriage and therapeutic abortion is associated with an increased likelihood of mother-to-child transmission (Hankins *et al*, 1993).

It is now thought that transplacental infection occurs shortly before, or at the time of, delivery. Labour and delivery are believed to be the times when the fetus is at greatest risk of becoming infected (Newell, 1993). The International Twin Registry also bears this out.

Of the 148 sets of twins that have been followed up, the evidence shows that Twin I is more likely to be infected than Twin II, with an odds ratio of 2.8. These figures demonstrate that birth is likely to be a time of transmission, with Twin I, the first to encounter the vaginal secretions, being more at risk than the second, who also has the benefit of two quantities of amniotic fluid to douche the vagina prior to his or her journey through the birth canal. Prematurity is also associated with a high risk of transmission. The earlier the gestation the greater the risk (European Collaborative Study, 1992).

Effects of HIV on the developing fetus

There is no evidence that HIV has any detrimental effects on the development of the fetus. Ultrasound examinations do not demonstrate any evidence of fetal anomalies or intrauterine growth retardation. There is some linkage between HIV infection and low birthweight, but this is probably due more to population differences, small sample sizes and intercurrent factors such as maternal intravenous drug use. Some studies have demonstrated an increase in spontaneous abortion and stillbirth rates, but these have not been generally replicated, and again may reflect the socioeconomic status of the mother than the effect of the disease.

Decision to continue with or to terminate the pregnancy

Clinicians have noted that many women who are aware of their HIV positive status decide to continue with their pregnancy. There are of course many factors involved in making the decision, including knowledge of transmission rates and the effect that pregnancy may have on disease progression, the current disease status of the women, as well as a host of other social and economic factors. In 1988 in Scotland, Johnstone et al reported that the women who continued with their pregnancy despite knowledge of the HIV status cited the following reasons: current good health; desire for a child; anti-abortion feelings; and knowledge of other women with HIV who had healthy children. Some women did cite HIV as a primary factor for choosing to terminate the pregnancy, but many said that social factors were equally important. In a study conducted in Paris between 1989 and 1992 (Mandelbrot et al, 1993), from a cohort of 289 women, 54 per cent elected to terminate their pregnancy and 46 per cent to continue with it. Demographic details were similar in both groups, and there was no difference in terms of age, transmission route, overall obstetric history, drug use, and clinical HIV status. Those women who had already had one or more children since diagnosis of their seropositivity were more likely to choose to terminate the pregnancy. Similarly, women who had already had an affected child were also more likely to terminate. However, women who had already undergone termination of pregnancy since their HIV diagnosis were more likely to continue with their pregnancy. It appears that the women's perception of the risk of having an infected child is the main determinant for choosing to terminate. The desire to have a child appears to outweigh medical and social factors for those women who have not delivered a child since their diagnosis.

OBSTETRIC INTERVENTIONS

Current research is focusing on interventions to reduce perinatal transmission. Interest centres on chemotherapy in pregnancy and interventions in labour.

Chemotherapy

The use of drugs in pregnancy is geared to the reduction of viral load in the mother, hoping that this will reduce the risks of mother-to-child transmission. In pregnancy the role of anti-retroviral therapy such as Zidovudine (AZT) has been under discussion. AZT has been used for some time in the management of HIV disease outside of pregnancy, but has unfortunately not been shown to be helpful in extending life expectancy (Concorde Study, Lancet 1993) or in decreasing the mother-to-child transmission rate. All drugs used in the management of AIDS have many very unpleasant side-effects, and only one, AZT, has been used in pregnancy. Maternal tolerance is limited as reported side-effects include anaemia, leucopenia, nausea and vomiting, fatigue and myopathy. Trials are still on-going about its safety in respect of teratogenicity, but to date there are no reported abnormalities from retrospective human studies. In animal studies there are no reports of fertility impairment, and the only abnormalities seen occurred when doses far in excess of normal were given to the animals (Sperling *et al*, 1992).

AZT has not seemed to be very effective in reducing mother-to-child transmission, but has not until recently been the subject of any trials. The AIDS Clinical Trial Group (ACTG) 076 study is studying the efficacy, safety and tolerance of AZT in prevention of vertical transmission. In March 1994, some preliminary results were released of a multicentre, double-blind, randomized, controlled trial using AZT in women who did not have any clinical indications for retroviral therapy, which gave a transmission rate of 8.3 per cent when both mothers and babies received AZT compared with a rate of 25.5 per cent when mothers and babies received placebo. AZT was commenced between 14 and 34 weeks gestation and given daily during pregnancy and labour, babies being given AZT within 24 hours of birth for six weeks (Roberts, 1994). This has important implications for reducing the mother-to-child transmission rate and is an exciting development. However, concerns about the possibility of long-term toxicity still need to be removed.

Interest is also centred on the newer anti-retroviral non-nucleoside-reverse-transcriptase-inhibitor (NNRTI) drugs that are available: TIBO and Nevirapine. NNRTIs also act upon reverse transcriptase stopping it from acting upon the RNA to change it to DNA, thus preventing replication of the virus. These drugs have their maximum effect within 24 hours, causing a rapid fall in level of the HIV p24 antigen. Unfortunately to date it has been demonstrated that the virus is able to develop resistance rapidly to these drugs. As the greatest risk of transmission appears to be close to the time of delivery, and the efficacy of the NNRTIs is limited to a short period before resistance occurs, it is thought that NNRTIs given in labour and in the first few weeks postpartum may both reduce the viral load at time of delivery, and the replication of any virus in the newborn. Studies using Nevirapine are being carried out currently in which the drug is given in labour and to both mother and baby for one week postpartum. This will theoretically reduce the viral load in labour, and also in the colostrum, and prevent replication of any virus that has passed from the mother to the fetus (Lange, 1993; Boucher, 1993).

Many physicians currently recommend that if AZT is to be used, it is used from the second trimester of pregnancy, when the risk of any teratogenicity is lower. It is thought that a combination of AZT and an NNRTI close to term for those who develop a resistant strain of virus may be helpful in the improvement in efficacy of the drugs, in the reduction of toxicity and the prevention of resistance, and possibly in reducing the vertical transmission rate.

Passive immunisation with Hyperimmune-immunoglobulin and monoclonal antibodies

In vitro studies have demonstrated that there are different types of virus, broadly divided into two, those causing a rapid disease progression and associated with a high transmission risk, and those associated with a slow disease progression and a low transmission risk. Women with the former are more likely to transmit the virus to their fetus. These mothers often had reduced antibody response to the virus. It is thought that passive immunisation of both mother and child in pregnancy with hyperimmune-immunoglobulin (HIVIg), from the latter type of virus, may help to reduce mother-to-child transmission in this group of women. There may be problems with the availability of such immunoglobulins, as it is estimated that it would require 500 donors to achieve the 10g of globulin required for one mother-child pair. There has been concern over the possible introduction of other antibodies with the HIVIg, but to date the trials conducted have not shown passive immunisation to be harmful (Rossi, 1993).

Vaccination with monoclonal antibodies has also been examined with a view to reducing mother-to-child transmission. In some studies such vaccination has decreased p24 antigen levels, decreased plasma viral RNA levels, raised antibody titres, and increased the CD4 count. One study used vaccination with one of the HIV proteins gp160 in post-HIV exposure subjects. It did not accelerate disease progression, and increased CD4 counts were observed. If AZT is combined with vaccination, the effects of the raised CD4 counts are increased. Other studies using gp160 in asymptomatic HIV patients have demonstrated improved immune responses. In the USA a study of maternal vaccination is planned to determine the effect on maternal disease and mother-to-child transmission. It is hypothesized though, that to be an effective form of intervention to reduce mother-to-child transmission, vaccination should be given prior to pregnancy, with a booster dose given during pregnancy (Wahren, 1993).

Interventions in labour

With the greatest risk of transmission occurring at time of delivery, interest has focused on interventions in labour which may reduce transmission. The interval between rupture of the amniotic membranes and delivery, and the duration of the second stage of labour may influence the transmission risk because of the exposure of the baby to HIV-infected body fluids. Uterine contractions may cause a leakage of maternal blood into the fetal circulation, and this effect may be exacerbated if the labour is prolonged. Trauma either to mother or fetus will increase the chance of blood-to blood contact.

Ascending infection from the birth canal to the fetus may occur in labour as a result of cervical dilatation and rupture of membranes. In addition, infection may occur from contact with, and inhalation and ingestion of, infected cells, amniotic fluid and maternal body fluids by the fetus as it negotiates the birth canal.

Given these risks, it has been suggested that HIV positive women should not be exposed to a long or difficult labour. The membranes should be left intact, and there should be a minimum of intervention where possible (Lefevre, Lepage, and Ravina, 1993). Internal continuous fetal electronic monitoring should be avoided, and where possible instrumental deliveries or episiotomies should not be performed.

Mode of delivery

There has been a debate about the use of caesarean section as the most appropriate mode of delivery in the prevention of intrapartum transmission. Several studies (European Collaborative Study, 1992; Villari *et al*, 1993) have demonstrated a trend towards a protective effect of elective caesarean section. It is thought that transmission may be reduced by avoidance of the route through the birth canal by the baby. There has been no randomized controlled trial showing a significant reduction in transmission, and indeed such a trial would have ethical implications, as the procedure is not without risk.

Performing a caesarean section may not reduce transmission if the infection has already been transmitted during the antenatal period. It would only reduce transmission in late-transmitting mothers. Currently there is not sufficient evidence to prove this or that the benefits of the procedure outweigh the drawbacks. Caesarean sections pose obstetric and non-HIV-related threats to both mother and child. Tovo (1993) comments that 16 HIV-infected women need to deliver by caesarean section to prevent one case of perinatal infection. It also presents a significantly increased risk to the team performing the procedure, although this should not be used as a reason to avoid the procedure when it is indicated.

Vaginal Lavage

Lavage of the birth canal has been suggested as an alternative method of reducing the risk of intrapartum transmission. Topical antiseptics have been used in labour for the prevention of neonatal morbidity in instances of maternal group B streptococcus infection. For use in the prevention of HIV transmission, the antiseptic agent must inactivate the virus both in vitro and in vivo, and must not cause any local or systemic toxicity. It must also be easy to prepare and use, and maintain a cost-effectiveness (Mandelbrot, 1993). There is only one antiseptic agent commercially available which fulfils all these criteria: benzalkonium chloride. Mandelbrot has suggested that the lavage of the birth canal should be repeated several times throughout labour.

The agent is introduced into the vagina via a speculum. This straight-forward procedure is therefore practicable throughout the world. There have been questions raised about the potential effects on the fetus of contact with the antiseptic agent, especially if inhaled or ingested, and as with any new development this procedure should be adequately tested prior to being universally advocated.

THE EFFECT OF PREGNANCY ON HIV

In the early 1980s when the disease was first diagnosed, it was noted that women who had given birth to babies who were subsequently diagnosed as having AIDS, themselves became ill and died. It was believed that the immunosuppressive effect of pregnancy caused the deterioration in the women's' condition. This was prior to the HIV antibody test, and the diagnosis was based on the baby's condition not the mother's positive test. It was not known how long the mother had been infected prior to her pregnancy. At the time it appeared that the pregnancy had acted as a factor in the mother's development of AIDS.

Prospective studies have since been performed, looking at the effects of pregnancy in terms of disease progression. MacCallum in Edinburgh in 1988 found that pregnancy did not cause a deterioration in the woman's health or immune system. Schoenbaum (1988) and Zamora (1993) also demonstrated this. The women in these studies were in good health at the time of their pregnancy, their immune system was not compromised.

A woman who is demonstrating signs of disease progression at the onset of her pregnancy, i.e. falling CD4 counts and incidents of opportunistic infections, may be affected by the immunosuppressive effect of pregnancy, and her CD4 count may be further lowered. It is still unclear whether terminating the pregnancy would influence this more rapid disease progression (Minkoff, 1987). Disease progression within pregnancy also poses a problem for treatment in respect of drugs and teratogenicity. Few drugs have been tested for use in pregnancy.

CHAPTER 5

Testing for HIV in Pregnancy

In 1985, HIV antibody testing became available, and thus the possibility of women discovering their HIV status prior to, or during pregnancy. Antenatal HIV testing has become an issue clouded by seemingly conflicting interests. Should a test be offered to every antenatal woman, to gain knowledge of the prevalence of the disease within the population, and to help improve the outcome for her baby? Or is the pregnant woman, who is already vulnerable, being exploited because she happens to be a useful 'subject' to study? There are many issues involved here, and it is helpful to understand some of the facts before recommendations are made.

What to test?

There is now available a range of tests with the ability to detect both the virus antibody and antigen.

Antibody testing is an indirect form of testing, detecting the antibody response to the infection. This is proof then of the presence of infection rather than the virus itself. It can take three months for these antibodies to form, so this form of testing will not identify those people in the window period between infection and antibody response. The benefit of this test is its reliability, with sensitivity and specificity levels approaching 99.5 per cent, therefore producing a very low false positive or negative rate. It is also an inexpensive test and is a good yardstick measure when used over a period of time. The most commonly used test is the Enzyme-Linked ImmunoSorbent Assay test (ELISA). HIV antigens are attached to a plastic sheet and the blood serum sample is added. If the sample contains antibodies, these will bind to the antigens. An anti-antibody is then added which will combine with the antigen-antibody complex. This has been labelled with an enzyme which will cause a colour reaction in the presence of a specific chemical. If the sample contains HIV antibodies, it will have bound to the sheet of HIV antigens, and the anti-antibody will have bound to this complex. When the chemical substrate is added a colour will form from the reaction with the enzyme bound anti-antibody.

In recent years, tests directly detecting the presence of the viral antigens have been developed. One of the antigens on the surface of the virus, the p24 antigen, can now be identified. However, the P24 antigen may not be detected in infants, and so this will not overcome the problem of identifying whether the baby is infected or carrying his or her mother's antibodies. Research on culturing the virus in vitro is continuing, but is difficult and expensive and has not yet to be proven to be reliable and consistent.

The latest and most reliable form of direct testing is the polymerase chain reaction (PCR) test. From a sample of blood the virus gene can be amplified in vitro and the DNA examined indicating the presence of infection. It is a complex test, and currently quite expensive. Pharmaceutical firms are marketing the test in kit form in order to simplify its use and to reduce the costs so that it can be used successfully in pathology laboratories worldwide. Inevitably, the dilemma will arise over the need for a diagnosis versus the expense entailed. Initial trials have shown the test to be accurate and reliable, moreover it can be used to test the blood of infants born to HIV positive mothers and enable a more rapid definition of their HIV status. However, the extreme sensitivity of the PCR test renders it prone to contamination from other samples, and exceptional standards are required of the laboratory, preferably a room dedicated to this function. Such facilities may not be possible in the developing world.

How to test?

There are two types of screening which may be used according to the intention of the programme. If prevalence monitoring is the aim, anonymous and unattributable testing can be used. The test result cannot be linked to the person, so information gained concerns the population tested rather than the individual. This presents an ethical problem in that there may be unidentified individuals who have been shown to be positive, and for whom no treatment or care can be given, and who may be unaware of their status.

Attributable testing, where the result can be linked to the individual, may be either named, or anonymous where the individual may give a false name or be identified by a number, initials, or code. This type of testing is intended to enable the individual to receive appropriate care and advice. To maintain ethical integrity the test must be of benefit to the individual in terms of his or her welfare, and the issues involved with the knowledge of HIV status be thoroughly explored and acknowledged by the individual prior to testing.

HIV test counselling

Any person undergoing an HIV test should have access to counselling both before and after the test. This is important because HIV infection is lifelong and life threatening. HIV infection affects a person's family life, sexual, work and social life, his or her spiritual and educational needs, legal status and civil rights. The term 'counselling' presumes that there will an exploration and clarification of the issues facing the woman, with a right to refuse the test, if this is the outcome of the discussion.

Pre-test counselling

The implications of having the virus or being at risk of contracting it, are manifold and involve all facets of life. It is important for the individual to have time to work through these concerns, to recognize how a diagnosis of HIV infection would affect each area, and to identify what support is required, and from where it will come.

The aims of this counselling are listed below.

- To provide information about the test itself, how it is performed, how long it will take for the results, and what the result means.

- To explore the implications of a positive result. Most people undergoing testing hope for, and expect, a negative result. It is necessary to explore how they would cope if the result were positive and who they would tell about it. The effects on the person's relationships, and possibly on his or her work should also be discussed.

- To promote health education and to identify and change behaviours which may have put the individual at risk. Guidance on safer sex, condom use, and needle exchange and usage may minimize further risk, irrespective of whether the individual actually has the test or not. It can also reduce the likelihood of infection or transmission to others.

- To assess the risk of exposure of the individual to HIV, giving the person time and opportunity to explore the reasons why they feel the test is indicated, or why it may have been suggested.

The assessment of risk "is a shaky tool, an inexact probe for an inexact science." (Sherr, 1991). The difficulty in categorizing behaviours or people is that there will be overinclusion of those who appear to have risk factors, and yet those who may be infected but who do not fit into any specific group may be missed. There are also cultural factors involved. For example, in Europe, intravenous drug use is a major risk factor, whereas in Africa this is seldom a problem. There are factors which are accepted as being universally risky.

- Frequency and type of sexual behaviour (including the partner's behaviour); specific sexual practices, in particular, high-risk practices such as vaginal and anal intercourse without the use of condoms, unprotected sexual relations with prostitutes. Unprotected sex with persons from sub-Saharan Africa is also included.

- Being part of a group with known high prevalence of HIV infection or with known high-risk lifestyles. For example, users of intravenous drugs, male and female prostitutes and their clients, prisoners, and homosexual and bisexual men. It is important to note that this is a very difficult and sensitive issue to raise, and especially in the antenatal clinic setting. Women may not be aware that their partners are bisexual, and many homosexual men report sexual encounters with women.

- Having received a blood transfusion, organ transplant, or blood or body products.

- Having been exposed to possibly non-sterile invasive procedures, such as tattooing and scarification.

It is important not to take the individual's knowledge about HIV and risk behaviour for granted. The risk factors may need exploring. It is equally important not to worry the individual unnecessarily, risk behaviour does not indicate the presence of infection.

Post-test counselling
Each person undergoing a test should receive post-test counselling.

The content of this will depend upon the outcome of the test, which may be a positive result, a negative result, or an equivocal result. It is good practice for test results to be given in person. It is a very tense time, and when bad news has to be given, it is advisable for there to be someone to offer support. It is also essential to have one system regardless of result to avoid the result being known 'by default', i.e. only those with positive results are called back to the clinic. Centres offering testing have developed protocols for giving results. Results are now rarely given on a Friday, when there are few agencies available over the weekend to give support, although if there is a good support network of family, the weekend may be appropriate, with useful time off available for coming to terms with the result.

Counselling following a negative result should include discussion about the window period. If it is three months or more since the last possible exposure to HIV, there is more certainty about the result. Prevention of further exposure must be explained, and the individual given the information to enable him or her to make choices about future safe behaviour. It is important to use the opportunity to encourage behaviour change and to ensure that the individual realizes that this is not just a 'reprieve'.

Counselling following a positive result must include time for the person to absorb the news. As with the giving of any bad news, reactions will vary from individual to individual. There is often a desire for factual information about the illness, treatment and prognosis. There may be a need for repetition of information as shock can often block comprehension. Response to the news will vary and depend on many physical and psychological factors which will be discussed later. A strategy for care and management needs to be agreed with the individual, which includes a plan for those whom he or she can involve and turn to for support.

An equivocal result may indicate that there has been a reaction with one of the non-HIV proteins, or that full seroconversion has not yet occurred. Counselling involves the giving of this information and the possible options. These include repeating the test (usually in a different laboratory, with three different ELISA tests), or to leave the test for a further three months to exclude the window period. The client will need considerable support in this time to cope with the stress that this delay will cause. Information about protection from further exposure from, and transmission to, others during this period must be given.

Why test?

HIV remains a relatively new disease. Information about spread, transmission and life expectancy is still limited. Testing programmes can be seen to benefit health by aiding research, gaining information about prevalence and spread within populations, and by assessing appropriate interventions.

When testing is considered, the benefits and harm must be clearly evaluated, whether group or individual, and informed consent gained. The purpose and gains must be clearly understood, as well as the possible sequelae for the individual. Curtis (Edinburgh, 1993) said, "Testing can be valuable for research, but there is limited evidence about its effectiveness for HIV prevention. Debate sometimes focuses on clinical benefits of testing while down-playing the emotional and social aspects."

The gaining of epidemiological data is often cited as one of the benefits of testing for HIV. The antenatal population appears to be an excellent target group to elicit such information. The vast majority are heterosexual, have been sexually active by definition, and form a cross-section of the entire population. In addition, they all have blood taken for routine antenatal investigations, thus facilitating the collection of the samples. However, they are not typical of the general population in as much as they are likely to be within a stable relationship, and therefore have fewer partners than the general non-pregnant population may have, and they have all had unprotected sex which may have altered their risk factors. The gathering of epidemiological data does not generally benefit the individual, and so must be questionable in the context of antenatal named testing.

The prevention of vertical transmission is also cited as a reason for testing women antenatally. This needs to be examined carefully. Previous chapters have discussed mother-to-child transmission, and current knowledge. It is not yet known exactly how or when the virus is transmitted transplacentally. With global rates of antenatal transmission ranging from 12 to 40 per cent, the only sure way to prevent transmission is to terminate the existing pregnancy and to avoid future pregnancies. The logical implication of terminating a pregnancy because of an HIV diagnosis is that all future pregnancies should also be terminated, with, for primigravid women, the reality of a renunciation of motherhood. There is no evidence to suggest that testing in pregnancy has resulted in a reduction of perinatal transmission (Sunderland *et al*, 1988). As discussed previously, many seropositive women continue with their pregnancies, and even go on to have further children. For many women, the need to fulfil their motherhood role is the deciding factor, and a decision to terminate or avoid pregnancy has to include alternatives to this role.

The prevention of vertical transmission by avoidance of breastfeeding is an important factor in advocating testing in the antenatal period. It would seem logical to protect the baby from this danger, especially if he or she had not been infected in utero or at delivery. However, this also needs to be evaluated in terms of geographical location, and an assessment made of relative risks in advocating alternative methods of infant feeding. This is further examined in Chapter 8.

It can be argued that women have a right to the information and to be able to make a choice. However, many women have said that they do not want to think about the issue of HIV whilst they are pregnant. "It is unnatural for human beings to know, before any symptoms appear, that they will develop a particular disease which is likely to kill them. Choosing not to know is a valid and meaningful coping strategy. Being tested is irrevocable, but a decision not to be tested always remains provisional." (Curtis, 1993).

The Department of Health (1992) has recommended that additional testing sites are created to offer the test to all women receiving antenatal care in higher prevalence areas, as there may be clinical benefits to the mother and her child of knowing their serostatus:

> ...evidence now suggests that an infected person may benefit clinically from prophylactic treatments to delay the onset of HIV related disease and from earlier treatment of any such conditions. Therefore testing for HIV infection can benefit both the individual and the public health.

The recommendation is for a diagnosis to be made early in the pregnancy, when the woman and her partner will have time to consider the options of termination of pregnancy, and care after the birth, such as breastfeeding. As discussed previously, many women choose not to opt for termination, and many would question the emotional suitability of discovering their diagnosis during pregnancy. It may give women and their partners an opportunity to consider adoption or fostering, which may be a useful option if their social circumstances are difficult. Testing does give the opportunity for those women who were unaware of the risks of transmission to be counselled on how to avoid transmission by safe practice.

One of the main arguments for testing in the antenatal period is to be able to plan more effectively the care that will be required by the neonate and its mother. It is now possible to detect the virus in the infant, to monitor the disease progression, and to initiate correct treatment. However the Concorde trial (Lancet, 1994) has shown that the use of AZT to delay onset of HIV related disease is not as effective as had been hoped, and that its effectiveness is of limited duration. There are still no treatments available to combat the progression of the disease effectively, and most of the drugs available have not been tested for safe use in pregnancy. It is important to note, as previously described, the use of AZT and Nevaripine within pregnancy, especially at the time of delivery may be useful in preventing mother-to-child transmission. Knowledge of HIV status can also lead to the avoidance of invasive procedures at the time of delivery, and breastfeeding postnatally.

Antibody testing of neonates may be seen differently from testing of antenatal women. The information is the same: whether the *mother* is carrying the virus or not. The focus is, however, on the well-being of the baby, and has a different psychological significance. It may be a useful option for those women who do not wish to be tested whilst pregnant.

Testing has been used as an opportunity for health promotion. Counselling can include information about risk behaviour, safer sex practices and prevention of transmission. A test, whether the result is positive or negative, can give the individual the opportunity to review their behaviour and change it if necessary. Even if the individual declines the test, the pre-test counselling can effect change in behaviour. In the light of the above discussion, this factor may be seen as the most positive outcome of HIV testing, especially in the antenatal period.

The biggest problem with one-off HIV antibody testing is the knowledge gained from the result. A negative result indicates that the individual is seronegative at the time of testing; it does not indicate if the individual has been infected but has not yet seroconverted. In addition, for some individuals, this ambiguity can lead to on-going concern about their status, and an obsession with being tested every three months, a group who have come to be known as the 'worried well'. A repeated negative test at three months, in the absence of repeated risk of exposure, will give a definite result. Conversely, for some individuals who may have put themselves at risk of contracting the virus in the past but who are not currently at risk, a negative test may end months or years of worry.

Testing positive at any time creates a major crisis within an individual. To be diagnosed whilst pregnant, and to have to cope with the implications of having a life-threatening infection and the significance this holds for her child and her family, creates for many an intolerable burden.

CONFIDENTIALITY

In many countries worldwide, there is a stigma attached to having HIV infection. Indeed, many countries deny entry to HIV positive individuals, and deport non-citizens. For many people there is active discrimination (employment, housing, insurance) if their HIV diagnosis is known. In the UK, being tested for HIV, irrespective of result, can lead to insurance and mortgages being denied. The social stigma is also very great, with HIV positive individuals often being shunned or rejected by their families and subject to abuse.

The United Kingdom Declaration of the Rights of People with HIV and AIDS includes among its rights the right to privacy. It goes on to say:

> we believe that information about the HIV status of any person should be confidential to that person and their appointed health and social carers...Information should not be disclosed to a third party about a person's HIV status without that person's consent.

In the UK, Genito-Urinary Medicine clinics have confidentiality guaranteed by law. This is not true of other clinics or health care settings. General Practitioners are required to divulge to insurance companies any medical condition which may have an impact on the policy applied for. The access to patient records within a general practitioner's surgery is not limited to the doctors, and pathology results are frequently left on clips or in trays awaiting the doctor's scrutiny.

All potential blood donors are asked to exclude themselves from donation if they have participated in risk activities as outlined previously. All blood donated is tested for HIV, and the result of this test, if positive, is usually sent to the donor's GP. Blood Transfusion Centres may also contact the donor themselves, and ask them to visit. The reason for the visit may not be apparent until the donor arrives. There has therefore been no pre-test counselling, no time for preparation or adjustment, and no support network prepared.

The fear associated with HIV has caused a potent reaction in every sphere - political, social, religious and medical. The fear of infection resulted in people with HIV infection being isolated physically and metaphorically. The medical world reacted to protect its workers and patients. Isolation procedures, 'danger of infection' stickers, and body bags took on a whole new meaning. Even though the diagnosis may not have been overtly stated, it was clearly apparent to all. Confidentiality is not easily maintained under those conditions.

The issue of whether and where to record the diagnosis is a contentious one. Many people have access to a patient's records within a hospital setting: doctors, nurses, midwives, physiotherapists, radiographers, radiologists to name a few. Should the result be recorded? Should the risk behaviour be noted? Should there be a code to record it discreetly? Who needs to know if a test has been performed and what the result is? Many practitioners would feel more comfortable by knowing the diagnosis. Logically speaking, practitioners are aware of the other diagnoses of their clients. Why should the spectre of HIV be continued by the omission of this diagnosis? It has long been accepted that the prevalence of HIV is unknown, and that HIV is no respecter of persons. Individuals may not realize that they have put themselves at risk.

Therefore, the only practical, non-discriminatory and safe way to practise is to employ 'universal precautions', i.e., all body fluids managed by the same, safe method.

If this was the case, then why should the result need to be recorded? HIV disease is most commonly managed by specialists is genito-urinary medicine. As stated previously, confidentiality is guaranteed within this setting. The advice that is given to their clients is that if treatment is required from another specialism, the diagnosis is disclosed on a 'need to know' basis. A woman who is HIV positive and who is pregnant, or contemplating pregnancy will become involved with the maternity services. From her obstetric perspective there may be no need to inform the obstetrician or midwife of her diagnosis, because she may need no special care within her pregnancy, and by the implementation of safe practice she is not putting the staff at risk. It would, however, be recommended that she did inform her named midwife and an obstetrician because of antenatal interventions that may be beneficial to the baby, such as drug therapy, and for the management of her labour. The choice would be hers, though. It would also be recommended for the paediatrician to be informed in order to prepare the management of the neonate.

Many people have suffered from breaches of confidentiality within the health care settings. Some of these have occurred as a result of attempts at discretion such as the use of codes or marking of notes in some way. The meaning of these is easily discovered, and not only discloses the diagnosis, but also draws one's attention to it. Others have occurred through fear and ignorance.

The Code of Professional Conduct drawn up by the United Kingdom Central Council for Nursing, Midwifery and Health Visiting (UKCC) states:

> As a registered nurse, midwife or health visitor, you are personally accountable for your practice and, in the exercise of your professional accountability, must: ...protect all confidential information concerning patients and clients obtained in the course of professional practice and make disclosures only with consent...

Breaches of confidence are subject to professional disciplinary proceedings, and civil action.

CHAPTER 6

Health Care Workers

Safe Practice

HIV is a fragile organism, easily inactivated by normal domestic hygiene measures. Other diseases are much more contagious, and have a higher infectivity rate. Accidental inoculation with HIV positive blood is estimated to have a 0.3 per cent risk of infection compared to a risk of 30 per cent with the Hepatitis B virus (Communicable Disease Report, 1991). To date there have been 182 known cases of health care workers worldwide becoming infected with HIV. Of these, 64 are proven to be through direct contact with clients and patients; four of these cases are in the UK. This has been following needlestick injury or through contamination of damaged skin or mucous membranes. 'Possible occupational exposure' has been cited for 118 cases, six of which are in the UK (PHLS Aids Centre, 1993).

As previously discussed, there is no way of knowing an individual's HIV status by looking at them, assessing their risk, or, on occasions, even by testing them. The only safe, sure and non-discriminatory way of practising is to take protective measures appropriate to the level of risk.

It is important to assess what risk of infection an activity carries. Body fluids which have high concentrations of virus are blood, semen, vaginal secretions, and, at times, breast-milk. Although HIV may be present in tears, saliva, urine and liquor amnii, the low concentration renders these body fluids 'low risk'. However, if these fluids are contaminated with blood, they become 'high risk' fluids.

Table 6.1: Assessment of appropriate protective measures

Assessment of risk/ activity	Protection required
Social contact, e.g. booking, antenatal visit	Nil
Exposure to body fluids - controlled situation, e.g. venepuncture	Gloves
Exposure to body fluids - uncontrolled setting, e.g. delivery, cord-cutting	Gloves, protective eye wear, apron, plastic sleeves

If there is no risk of contact with body fluids, then there needs to be no protective measures taken. Intact, healthy skin is a good protection from the virus. Any skin diseases or lesions on the hands should be reported to the occupational health department, and advice sought about protective measures, such as the wearing of gloves. Any skin abrasion on exposed skin should be covered by an island plaster, and changed whenever required.

When gloves are worn these should be of vinyl or latex material, worn for single use and discarded. Hands should still be washed before and after wearing gloves to prevent the spread of microorganisms.

Protective clothing will only prevent contamination of exposed areas by splashes. It cannot protect the skin from puncture by sharps. Each practitioner is responsible for their own use and safe disposal of sharps. It has been demonstrated that operative procedures carry a high risk of glove puncture (Smith and Grant, 1990). It is important to practise safe techniques when using sharp instruments. Venepuncture and injections are the commonest procedures performed, and are associated with needlestick injuries. Equipment is now available to reduce the risk associated with venepuncture. Evacuated sample bottles and multisample needle holders are a system whereby sample bottles can be filled directly whilst the needle remains in the vein. The needle and holder are then discarded without any disconnection being required. This avoids the manipulations involved in transferring the blood from syringe to bottles. It is very dangerous to resheathe needles, and this should always be avoided. Sharps boxes should be of rigid plastic, resisting penetration by needles. They should always be replaced when they are two-thirds full, to avoid injury from depositing sharps into a full container.

The delivery of a baby has the potential for blood loss in an uncontrolled setting. It is good practice to protect against eye-splashes by wearing protective spectacles with side pieces, and skin exposure by wearing plastic sleeves. Material gowns do not prevent contact with blood. If these precautions are used at every delivery, it will become as common a practice as wearing gloves, and as acceptable to mothers and their partners.

The use of protective spectacles is as important during the repair of the perineum, as there is very likely to be splashes of blood, and the eyes are in closer proximity.

Accidents

If ungloved hands come into contact with blood, vaginal secretions, liquor, lochia or breast-milk, they should be washed with soap and water. Should a needlestick or puncture injury occur, first-aid measures of encouraging bleeding from the site, washing with soap and water, and covering with an occlusive dressing should be employed, and the incident reported to the occupational health department. The incident should also be reported to the person in charge, and an accident form completed. Some practitioners seek testing for HIV antibodies, this is discussed below.

If eye-splashes of blood or liquor occur, the eye should be irrigated with normal saline, 20 ml undines of normal saline should be available in the areas where such incidents are likely to occur.

Spillages of blood should be removed promptly and cleaned with hot water and detergent, and wiped with an hypochlorite solution.

Health Care Workers and HIV Infection

Blood-borne viruses are known to have been transmitted from health care workers to patients. There have been a number of outbreaks of Hepatitis B infection among patients operated on by doctors and dentists with acute infection, or who were HBe carriers. The same possibility exists with HIV, although the risk is considerably less than for Hepatitis B. To date there has only been one reported case worldwide of an infected health care worker who has transmitted the virus to a patient. The mode of transmission in this case remains unclear.

The Department of Health (1994) document, 'Guidance on the Management of Infected Health Care Workers' states:

> All other retrospective studies worldwide, of patients exposed to the potential risk of transmission of HIV during exposure prone invasive procedures have failed to identify any who become infected by this route. [Para. 2.3]

There is evidence that the risk of transmission of HIV from infected patients to workers is far greater, with 182 reported cases up to December 1993. (*Ibid.*)

Every health care worker has a professional and statutory duty to the patient to 'do no harm'. The UKCC Code of Professional Conduct states that each registered nurse, midwife and health visitor shall:

> Act always in such a way as to promote and safeguard the well being and interests of patients/clients.
> Ensure that no action or omission on his/her part or within his/her sphere of influence is detrimental to the condition or safety of patients/clients.

There is, therefore, an ethical duty to protect patients. The recommendations (see Appendix II) of the Department of Health document, 'Guidance on the Management of Infected Health Care Workers' states that those who believe they may have been exposed to infection with HIV in their personal life, or in the course of work, must seek medical advice and possibly diagnostic testing. Those found to be infected should not undertake exposure prone invasive procedures. Included in the definition of such procedures are:

- the surgical entry into tissues, cavities, organs or repair of major traumatic injuries;

- vaginal or caesarean deliveries, or other obstetric procedures during which sharp instruments are used.

The Expert Advisory Group on AIDS further clarified the position of an infected health care worker in obstetrics.

> Infected health care workers may safely participate in routine antenatal and postnatal care and perform non-invasive procedures such as ultrasound. When undertaking a vaginal delivery they must not perform procedures involving the use of sharp instruments such as the infiltration of local anaesthetic or the suturing of a tear or episiotomy. Neither can they participate in an instrument delivery requiring forceps or suction since these may need an episiotomy and subsequent repair. Therefore in practice, this means that an infected health care worker may only undertake a vaginal delivery if it is certain that a second midwife or doctor will also be present in the delivery room or home and able to undertake such operative interventions that might arise during the course of the delivery.

The implications of these statements are that the health care worker who has been at risk of contracting HIV must establish their diagnosis. This will be by an HIV antibody test. This may of course be performed at a genito-urinary medicine clinic. If the result is positive, the health care worker is then required to inform the occupational health department to seek advice about their work and practice. This disclosure of the diagnosis will have immediate effects within the work environment. Midwives and doctors are expected to be able to work in any situation. To remove a worker from a particular area, or to restrict his or her activity within that area is liable to raise questions and indicate the diagnosis. This means that whilst a patient's confidentiality is to be maintained at all times, a health care worker's may be breached by default, although there may have been no formal disclosure.

The duty of preserving the health care worker's confidentiality may conflict with the duty to inform patients who may have been at risk of infection. It may be necessary to explain the circumstances leading to the concern, but a disclosure of the worker's identity should only be made with consent, or in order to treat anxieties. Any such breach of confidentiality is required to be justified.

Many occupational health departments have an inoculation incident procedure. This includes the above advice regarding first aid and the reporting of the incident. It is common practice to test the patient's blood for Hepatitis B antigen, following consent. The health care worker's Hepatitis B status should be recorded in the records, as this is now a requirement of employment. This can be checked, the degree of contamination and the risk of infection assessed. HIV testing may be carried out:

- if the assessment concludes there is a significant risk of HIV infection;
- if informed consent has been obtained from the patient;
- when either the consultant occupational health physician, or in his or her absence, the consultant microbiologist has been consulted.

A sample of the health care worker's blood may be obtained and stored for three months, when a second sample will be obtained, and the two samples tested for HIV. This will establish the worker's status at the time of the incident. Irrespective of the result, the health care worker should receive counselling and support, and advice regarding prevention of further injury.

CHAPTER 7

Caring for a Woman with HIV in Pregnancy

PRACTICAL ISSUES

Pregnancy

The care that a woman receives in her pregnancy must be responsive to her needs. The woman with HIV disease requires all the usual care that any woman receives, and in addition has some special needs.

Named midwife and team working

The diagnosis of her seropositive status may have been made prior to, or during her pregnancy. The woman may have been in contact with specialist services, and have built up a rapport with the team caring for her. It is important that this rapport and liaison continues throughout the pregnancy.

The establishment of a small team of carers is very helpful. Johnstone (1992) recommends:

> multiagency care, easy and effective communication, an awareness and understanding of other issues (which may be more important to the mother than her HIV infection), and specialists with both experience and an up-to-date knowledge base.

This allows for seamless care, as the woman moves through her pregnancy to motherhood. The team should be comprised of the named midwife, the genito-urinary specialist, an obstetrician, a paediatrician, and a health visitor A social worker and drug worker may also need to be involved depending on the circumstances. The general practitioner may act as the link between the HIV, drug, antenatal and paediatric services. The midwife should, where possible, be experienced and knowledgeable about HIV disease, the support systems available, and the physical, psychological and material needs associated with such a diagnosis. It is equally important for the midwife to have his or her own support network, as it is very stressful caring for women with a potentially fatal disease (Brierley, 1993). It is useful if a midwife partnership can be established to both aid in continuity of care and to provide support for one another.

It is also important that the mother's care is coordinated with the ongoing care she receives for her HIV disease. Combination of clinic attendances should be arranged so that the mother is not duplicating visits. Some centres have organized family clinics, when affected children and parents can be seen together.

Counselling

The health promotion and education opportunity offered to a woman on her introduction to the maternity services may have been the catalyst for her diagnosis. It is clearly necessary for midwives to develop and be competent in the skills required for this initial pre-test counselling. This is especially so in areas of high prevalence, where the volume of women booking for maternity care exceeds the capacity of the specialist counsellors.

Some women seek counselling prior to conception, and consider the risks involved before embarking on the pregnancy. Where the woman is HIV negative with an HIV positive partner, the possibility of using donor sperm, or treated sperm of the partner should be raised and discussed.

The issues to be discussed in order for an informed choice to be made about having a child include the following:

- possible risk to the woman's health;
- the risk of vertical transmission;
- the possibility of the mother's illness or death during the baby's childhood;
- the prognosis of an infected child.

As previously discussed, a woman who is well and asymptomatic will find this difficult to imagine, and it is often other social and economic factors which are uppermost in her decision regarding the continuation of the pregnancy. Great sensitivity is required in helping the woman come to terms with her decision. She has the prospect of terminating her child, which may or may not have been infected, or continuing with the pregnancy with the worry of bearing an infected child, and of leaving the child motherless, if and when she herself dies.

HIV disease management

Women who are diagnosed with HIV during the pregnancy should undergo a thorough clinical examination to assess evidence of HIV infection. The following investigations should be performed:

- Full blood count
- Liver function tests
- CD4 count
- P24 antigen
- Hepatitis B antigen
- Toxoplasmosis serology
- Syphilis serology
- Cervical cytology
- Screening for STDs

(Mercey, Bewley and Brocklehurst, 1993).

For many women in the UK, HIV is transmitted sexually, and so screening for other sexually transmitted diseases (STD) should be performed as these will also affect the pregnancy outcome.

Tuberculosis is a problem in areas of the USA, especially New York, and in Africa. Malaria should also be excluded in women who are from areas where it is endemic. Immune-compromised women are also susceptible to toxoplasmosis and cytomegalovirus. Booking blood investigations should include screening for these infections.

Cervical dysplasia and neoplasia is a common manifestation of HIV among women (McCarthy *et al*, 1993). As it can progress rapidly in pregnancy, it is important that cervical screening is also performed.

The woman is monitored routinely every three months for disease progression, and efficacy of treatment, if initiated, and more frequently if there is evidence of significant immunosuppression. The markers of disease progression are laboratory tests and clinical assessment of symptoms.

Full blood count	Anaemia, lymphopenia, neutropenia, thrombocytopenia are associated with HIV infection, independently or together.
CD4 count	The CD4 count, although lowered by pregnancy, is a useful marker, and is used to indicate when prophylactic treatment should begin. It is agreed by clinicians that major opportunistic infections are unlikely to occur when the CD4 count is >300/mm^3. Prophylactic treatment is commenced if the CD4 count falls below 200/mm^3 (Johnstone, 1992). The CD4 count has a diurnal variation and should be measured at the same time of day.
P24 antigen	May be found at seroconversion, and with increasing immunosuppression. It may precede the onset of symptoms.

(Mercey, Bewley and Brocklehurst, 1993)

The clinical assessment may be complicated by the overlapping of signs and symptoms associated with HIV disease and those of pregnancy. Tiredness, nausea, vomiting, anaemia, and candidiasis are all common to both conditions. Oral candidiasis though, is associated with HIV disease, along with hairy leucoplakia.

Prophylaxis consists of prevention of the most common opportunistic infection, pneumocystis carinii pneumonia, by co-trimoxazole or aerosolized pentamidine. Co-trimoxazole is thought to be safe for use in pregnancy, with no evidence of harm noted by Briggs *et al* (1983). It also appears to have a prophylactic effect against toxoplasmosis. The effects of pentamidine in pregnancy are unknown, but aerosolized administration allows for little systemic absorption and is often given monthly.

Zidovudine (AZT) has been used in pregnancy (see Chapter 4), but its safety is not totally proven, and the drug is not licensed for use in pregnancy. The side effects also render it unacceptable to many people, especially added to the minor disorders of pregnancy. If used, AZT is avoided within the first trimester, to avoid the risk of teratogenicity. AZT is associated with anaemia, as is pregnancy, and so a full blood count should be performed regularly, and iron therapy initiated promptly if indicated.

Pregnancy management

Invasive procedures such as chorionic villus sampling and amniocentesis carry the risk of infecting the fetus by introducing maternal blood during the procedure. Parents may be anxious to know if the child the woman is carrying has been infected. HIV has been cultured from aborted fetuses at 8 weeks gestation. It is possible to culture the virus from fetal cells. However, the hazards of the procedure with the risk of introducing the virus to an uninfected fetus, and the risk of miscarriage need to be explained. There is also a risk of obtaining a false positive result from contamination of the fetal sample with maternal blood (Dick, 1992). More importantly, mother-to-child transmission may occur at any point in the pregnancy, and especially at the time of delivery. Screening in early pregnancy is therefore not reliable. Overall, it is advisable to avoid such procedures.

Other health-related problems which coexist need to be included in the antenatal management. Intravenous drug use has been a common route of infection, and the woman may need the help of drug agencies and support workers, to achieve control over her habit, and where possible to establish an oral dosage of methadone. Drug dependency is often associated with poverty, homelessness, and smoking. These all have a deleterious effect on fetal growth, and so this should be monitored regularly by ultrasound examination.

Labour and delivery

As discussed in Chapter 4, interventions in labour should be kept to a minimum. It is preferable for labour to commence spontaneously. The decision to induce a labour should be made according to the usual obstetric indications. It is important to avoid a long labour and subsequent intervention measures, and a caesarean section may be indicated if medical induction by the use of extra-amniotic oxytocin is not achieving onset of labour. It is preferable to avoid artificial rupture of membranes.

All forms of analgesia are suitable. The use of pethidine in drug-using mothers may not be effective. Very high doses are required for an analgesic effect, which may be prohibitive for the fetus. Epidural analgesia may be associated with a higher incidence of instrumental delivery, and should be used with caution. The policy of permitting a long second stage allowing for descent and rotation prior to active pushing may overcome this problem.

Other invasive procedures such as internal fetal monitoring, fetal blood sampling and instrumental deliveries should be avoided as these have been linked with the increased possibility of transmission. However, clinical judgement about relative risks should be made. The risk to an asphyxiated baby of an instrumental delivery to expedite delivery may be less than the increased risk of transmission.

It is preferable to avoid episiotomy during delivery. A ventouse delivery may be achieved with an intact perineum, but the application of the cup to the scalp may cause more trauma than forceps.

Puerperium

The baby should be bathed following delivery to wash off any blood and liquor provided the room temperature is at least 23°C. Exclusions to this include: preterm and small for gestational age babies; babies who were distressed in utero or who required resuscitation following delivery; and babies who are unwell or whose temperature is below 36.5°C.

The postnatal care should be the same as for any other mother and baby. There is no need for a separate room, unless the mother is unwell and has a low CD4 count. In these circumstances, she is more at risk of being infected by others, and a separate room may afford her some protection. The baby of a drug-using mother may need special or intensive care, but otherwise mother and baby should remain together.

All mothers are encouraged to be as independent as possible post-delivery, and will usually be able to look after their own hygiene needs. Lochia should be treated as any other body fluid, and gloves worn when handling pads or examining the perineum. Detergent and paper towels should be made available for cleaning purposes in all bathrooms and toilets, and any blood spillages should be cleaned with a recognized agent such as Presept®.

Contraception

All mothers receive advice about contraception in the postpartum period. This usually concentrates on the prevention of pregnancy. For a couple, where one or both members has HIV infection, this must also include information about prevention of infection. This advice must also be given in the pre- and post-test counselling as pregnant women continue to have unprotected sex as the risk of pregnancy no longer applies.

Compared with other sexually transmitted diseases such as gonorrhoea, HIV is poorly transmitted via sexual intercourse. Some people can have unprotected intercourse many times without becoming infected, others though, may be infected after a single act (Johnson, 1988). It appears that some people are more infectious than others, and some are more susceptible to infection than others (Bury, 1989). Some sex workers have remained HIV negative despite undergoing the same risks as their colleagues who have seroconverted.

Couples who are both HIV positive may assume that there is no need to protect themselves from infection. However, they may both re-infect the other risking an accelerated progression of their disease. In addition, should the virus have been contracted from a previous partner, they are at risk of contracting a different strain of virus, which may be more virulent. Barrier methods, then, should always be used.

Prevention of pregnancy and HIV infection

The *combined oral contraceptive pill* has been shown to suppress the immune system, but not in as great a measure as pregnancy itself. There are no contraindications to its use in HIV, other than existing liver damage, which may be present in drug-users who have had hepatitis.

The *progestogen only pill* does not affect liver function and is entirely suitable for use in women with HIV infection. The need to take the pill at a regular time every day may render it unsuitable for some women. The injectable form giving protection for three months is also available which may be more suitable for some women.

The *intrauterine contraceptive device* (or coil) is associated with an increased risk of pelvic infection, and as this can increase the risk of progression of HIV disease, this method has been not advised for use in HIV infection. However, Mercey, Bewley and Brocklehurst (1993) state that: "there is no evidence of an extra risk of pelvic inflammatory disease in HIV-infected coil-users." There may also be increased risks of viral transmission because of the heavier vaginal discharge and heavier periods associated with the coil, which will increase the number of HIV infected cells within the vagina (Bury, Morrison and McLachlan, 1992).

Some *barrier methods* may afford some protection from HIV as well as pregnancy. The exact method of transmission from semen to the female blood stream is not understood. If this occurs in the cervix, a cervical barrier may afford some protection, but if it occurs in the vagina it will not. Similarly it is not known whether the male becomes infected from vaginal or cervical secretions. The diaphragm or cap combined with a spermicide containing nonoxynol-9 may be effective protection against both pregnancy and HIV, but there are no studies which support or discount this.

The *male condom* is the commonest and most reliable protection against infection and pregnancy. However, the condom is only reliable as long as it is used correctly. Latex is impermeable to HIV, and condoms are manufactured to stringent standards. In practice condoms do burst or leak, and careless removal and damage by oil-based lubricants render the condom unsafe. A leading condom manufacturer is at present developing a polyurethane condom which may overcome these problems. Many men are reluctant to use condoms, thus reducing the woman's ability to protect herself, and condom use depends upon male arousal. The *female condom* has recently been released on the market. It is made from polyurethane which is much stronger than latex, and is resistant to the passage of HIV. The woman can retain control over her protection, and it does not rely on male arousal. The polyurethane is also less likely to be damaged by oil-based lubricants and creams. The condom covers the labia thereby affording greater protection than the male condom. It is however less comfortable to use, and is considerably more expensive than the male condom.

Spermicides containing Nonoxynol-9 are an effective protection against HIV. Nonoxynol-9 has been shown to inactivate HIV in laboratory experiments. Condoms lubricated with Nonoxynol-9 do then have this extra protection if the condom breaks. However, Nonoxynol-9 is often reported by users to cause irritation of the genital tract lining, actually causing a greater risk of entry of any virus present.

PSYCHOLOGICAL ISSUES

The shadow of HIV can affect women long before they decide to consent to testing. Some women have worried about the possibility of being positive because they are aware of the risks to which they have been exposed. The reasons for being tested are many and varied: the need to know; having been exposed to a particular risk; a new partner; contemplating pregnancy; a response to symptoms. Some women have been unaware that they have been tested, e.g. blood donation, and have not seen themselves as having been at risk. Pre-test counselling aims to help individuals to identify how they will cope with a positive and a negative result. Behaviour change may be indicated whatever the result. If negative, to avoid a similar risk occurring again, if positive, to prevent reinfection and cross-infection.

Bisset and Gray, in 'Working with Women and AIDS' state that:

> Perhaps the most difficult and also the most fundamental question facing anyone considering being tested is whether the personal resources and social support network, necessary to survive and live with a positive result, are available. The knowledge of being infected may change the whole pattern of someone's life and shatter dreams for the future. Clearly the situation is even more complex for pregnant women who have to consider an unborn child. (Bury, Morrison and McLachlan, 1992).

It is very important for the woman to have prepared the coping strategies and support network she plans to use. People entering into a test usually do so with the expectation that it will be negative. A positive result is shocking and shattering. It may confirm worst fears, it may have dashed realistic hopes. It is a reality which cannot be changed or undone. The world of the future, plans and dreams has ended and another has begun, that of hospitals, clinics, blood tests, fear, hostility, stigma and death. It is often impossible for people to see any future with a positive diagnosis. At first, thoughts may turn to the reality of ultimate death, "I am going to die".

First reactions vary, but most follow the pattern of the grief process: numbness, shock, denial, anger. Many people on hearing their positive diagnosis are numb, and cannot hear what the counsellor is telling them. Information will not be absorbed. Some return to familiar coping strategies such as drug-taking or alcohol abuse. Another phase is denial, with the individual avoiding the support offered by the health services, with the hope that avoidance means the diagnosis it is not true.

This denial and avoidance can lead to a feeling of great isolation. Many people once diagnosed feel very lonely and very afraid. The spectre of their positivity is always present, colouring each day and every activity. The establishment of support groups has been of tremendous help to those affected by HIV, especially to those who are HIV positive, but also to their families, who may need help to support their loved ones. When HIV was first identified, the majority of people affected were men. The first women to be diagnosed felt very isolated. Although the support groups for men were helpful in respect of understanding how it felt to be infected, there was a need for a women's group.

> I met some gay men who were positive and that was great - a real relief to be able to talk about my fears around dying, and other such things. Yet it wasn't really enough - there were still so many issues not touched upon and concerns which we did not have in common. What I really wanted was to meet other HIV positive women I could talk to about my fears about having children - or rather not having children - about sex, relationships and so on. (Thomson, 1993)

Positively Women developed as a response to this need, and offers practical and emotional support to women with HIV, including group meetings, written information and a telephone helpline.

This feeling of isolation is compounded by the fear of telling people. This is a very understandable fear. People react in a variety of ways, many of which are not helpful. Families may reject the individual, and each person will have to undergo a similar grief process of shock, denial, anger and depression. A woman may be rejected by her partner, and be left alone and unsupported at the very time she needs him most. If she should also be pregnant this will be even more terrifying. Parents may fail to understand how the daughter feels, and may blame her for 'bringing this on them'. Friends may not be able to cope with the shock or prospect of supporting the woman through the experience. It is very difficult to offer the right kind of support when there is no understanding of the reality. If the person told is supportive and helpful, this can bring an enormous sense of relief, and decrease the sense of isolation.

Anger is another common manifestation, primarily about dying. It is often released in many directions, and at many people. There has been, and still is in some quarters, much ignorance, prejudice and stigmatization among officialdom which causes hurt and frustration. Anger can be hard to receive, and the midwife and other carers need to be able to understand the reasons, and allow expression of this anger. Repressed anger can lead to depression. Women can develop a low self-esteem and many blame themselves for becoming infected.

The end of the grief process is acceptance. Each individual will come to this at their own pace, and each stage may last differing periods of time, and may have to be revisited. Acceptance can lead to readjustment and reorganization of one's life. Women may decide on their own goals or achievements. They may become very ambitious to reach these, and use their diagnosis as a catalyst for achievement.

There may be an intense need for information and knowledge about HIV disease, and an overwhelming commitment to this. It is important that those with HIV are given precise and accurate information about the disease. They need to know how the virus is and is not transmitted. They need to know that there is no risk in social contact, in kissing and hugging their loved ones. Information gives the individual power and control, and when one's control over life has been removed it is important to give back as much control as possible.

A realization of one's mortality can raise huge issues about parenthood. Women who are childless may very seriously consider having a child. As the information available about HIV and pregnancy has developed and become available, so women with HIV have become more informed.

> It is not unusual for a person infected by HIV or AIDS and his/her partner or spouse to have an overwhelming desire to leave behind some creation, and a child symbolizes this need. A woman may regard becoming a mother as an important aspect of how she sees herself and her future, reinforced by societal influences. (Barlow, 1992)

For women with children, there is another fear, that of knowing whether their children are infected. It may be that their own diagnosis was made following that of their child's. It is a time of extreme tension, anxiety and guilt. They fear for their children's future, when they should be told their diagnosis, and how long they will live. For those who are, or who become pregnant, there is the decision to make regarding the continuation of pregnancy, with all the implications of that decision.

Women from ethnic minorities may have another set of problems to encounter. There may be cultural taboos around the subject of sex, information may be difficult for them to obtain, and control over information, access to health care, and their own protection may not be in their hands. The needs of these women may be misunderstood and they may become marginalized under the stronger influence of the 'majority' culture.

The range of feelings and needs of women with HIV is very wide and at times may be very difficult to keep up with. The support required involves non-judgmental listening to what each woman identifies as her need, and an interactive participation to enable the woman to think through her problems, for her to understand her responses and to identify helping strategies and solutions.

SOCIAL ISSUES

Many of the women affected by HIV will already be in a vulnerable position. Women are still subordinate to their male partners in many countries, and hold many and complex roles. Women are the main care-providers in the community, as mothers, daughters, partners and siblings. They are affected as well as infected.

> Women living with HIV in the community will usually bear the responsibility for child care, housekeeping, health .... appointments, *and* their own illness, as well as the illness of partner, possibly children and other family members. (Barlow, 1992)

This is true worldwide, women traditionally bear this burden without the attendant power to make decisions. Historically, HIV has been a male disease, and this has left women without the back-up and support services that have been created by and for their male counterparts. This is also borne out medically, where the medical problems specific to women have been ill-recognized and researched, and where drug trials favour problems common to both, e.g. for pneumocystis carinii pneumonia treatment and prophylaxis.

Women, then, will often be both carers and patients, and will need the support to be able do this. Many of the problems faced, e.g. housing, financial, health, all require appointments in different venues and involving different personnel. A link person acting as a liaison with different agencies can reduce time and effort, and coordinate the support. The introduction of family clinics with linked medical social workers will reduce the amount of travelling required, and speed up the requests for help.

In the UK, there has been a multidisciplinary initiative to examine the needs of women with HIV, and how these can be met. The following framework was devised through collaboration between women service users, women practitioners, managers from social services, health providers and voluntary organizations.

*Table 7.1: Principles to be included in planning care
(Cleary and Young, 1993)*

Principles to underpin provision of services	Needs to be considered when planning care
Equality	Information and advice
Consultation	Financial advice
Informed consent	Legal advice
Advocacy	Child care needs
Respect and dignity	Housing
Access to information	Home-based help
Service accessibiliy and availability	Respite care
Collaboration	Counselling
Coordination	Health needs and sexual health needs
User-involvement	Refugee & immgration status advice

Support groups also fulfil the role of informing women about what support is available and how to access it. More importantly, their existence is testimony to the fact that it is alright for women to need help, and that they are not alone.

CHAPTER 8

The Neonate

The neonate may or may not be infected by HIV from his or her mother, but will certainly be affected by HIV infection. Even if he or she is one of the 60-80 per cent who is not infected in pregnancy or delivery, the infection is likely to leave him or her motherless during childhood, and will affect every member of his or her family. If the mother's diagnosis is known in pregnancy, it will be an anxious time as she waits to know if the baby is infected, and watches for every sign that might indicate infection. For the medical carers there are the concerns of which test is most accurate, which treatment should be commenced, if there is any form of effective prophylaxis, which is the safest method of feeding, and how best to support the family. This chapter will focus on these issues.

Testing the neonate

At the delivery of a baby, the mother's first question is usually, "Is it a boy or a girl?", and the second question is, "Is he or she alright?". For a woman with HIV, this second question may not be answered for many months. The initial examination may show the baby to be clear of any obvious congenital anomalies, but the worry of whether the virus has been transmitted is not so easily allayed. An early diagnosis is clearly preferable for the mother, but is also essential for the correct management of the disease.

Until fairly recently, the only method of HIV detection was antibody testing. All newborns of HIV infected mothers will carry their mother's HIV antibodies. Babies would have to be tested regularly until the antibodies either disappeared (usually by 15-18 months) or were shown to remain, indicating that the baby had begun to manufacture his own antibodies, and was therefore infected by the virus.

With the introduction of the polymerase chain reaction (PCR), p24 antigen and virus isolation tests, it has become possible to diagnose

HIV infection by the age of six months. Individually these tests have not proven reliable for use in neonates. P24 antigen may not always be present in the neonatal period, and PCR may not always give a positive result. Garburg-Chenon *et al* (1993) report that 70 per cent of their sample of infants were repeatedly positive in PCR and antibody testing, whereas all had a positive viral culture, 73 per cent of seronegative children had negative PCR and in vitro antibody production tests. There were some children who were antibody negative, but who had one positive viral culture, and occasional positive PCR results. The authors recommend that a combination of viral culture, PCR and in vitro antibody production tests is performed to improve earlier detection. Perez-Alvarez *et al* (1992) also recommend a combination of tests, following their study in which they used four markers of infection: p24 antigen (which was present in 78 per cent of those infected; HIV culture, present in 75 per cent; HIV antibodies, present in 50 per cent; and specific determination of IgM antibodies, present in 92 per cent. These latter were also detected in 33 per cent of seronegative children. The authors conclude:

> The problems due to the low sensitivity in p24 antigen detection, HIV isolation and the detection of ... antibodies, as well as the low specificity of the IgM detection, means that it is necessary to simultaneously use several techniques in the diagnosis of children. (Perez-Alvarez *et al*, 1992)

Some of the tests mentioned are only available in well-equipped laboratories, and are expensive to perform. This excludes many of the under-developed countries. Bredberg-Raden *et al* (1993) reported that PCR showed a high specificity and sensitivity for early diagnosis in infants in their study in Tanzania. The p24 antigen assay and ELISA antibody test were also useful for diagnosis in infants, their specificity and sensitivity increasing after 8 weeks of life. These latter tests can be conducted in routine laboratories. In Italy, Caselli *et al* (1993) are developing a test based on the detection of HIV-specific IgG-3 antibodies. In their study, 39 out of 44 infants born to HIV positive mothers tested negative when tested at a median of day five of life. Of these children, 35 were confirmed as not infected. This gave a prediction rate of 89 per cent. The median age of a negative result was two months, as compared to 15 months using the ELISA test solely. The authors also claim that the test is comparatively simple, uses low-technology and is low-cost.

Table 8.1: Comparison of tests in neonatal and paediatric testing

Test Name	What it looks for	Benefits	Drawbacks
HIV Antibody	Antibodies, ie an indirect test	Good as a long-term marker Cheap Can be performed in routine laboratory	Not testing neonate, but mother, as it is the maternal antibodies which are initially detected; diagnosis of paediatric infection cannot be made until at least 15 months.
Polymerase Chain Reaction (PCR)	HIV Antigens, ie a direct test	Earlier detection of infection, by six months	High incidence of false negatives in neonates Expensive Needs special laboratory facilities
p24	HIV Antigen, ie a direct test	Early detection of HIV May be conducted in routine laboratory Sensitivity increases after 8 weeks of life	Not always present in neonates
IgM Antibodies	Specific antibody, ie indirect test	Useful auxiliary method	Poor specificity
IgG-3 Antibodies	Specific HIV antibodies	Early detection (5 days) Appears to be specific Claimed to be simple and low-cost	When used with ELISA (antibody test) can give earlier results Requires further studies

It is recommended that a combination of tests is used.

An early diagnosis of HIV infection in the postnatal period provides good opportunity for correct and active management of the disease. Where disease is acquired at delivery or postnatally, the diagnosis will be not be made in the neonatal period. Analysis of the success of the different methods of testing should take this into account.

It must be remembered that consent needs to be obtained for neonatal testing as for adults. The mother must be informed and give her consent, especially as in reality it is she who is being tested. If HIV antibodies, or antigens are detected it is proof of maternal infection. Where testing is indicated from clinical signs of HIV infection in the baby, and where the mother has not yet been tested, all the implications of testing and counselling needs should be explored for the mother as it is her diagnosis which is being tested too. The request and result must be treated with the same respect for confidentiality.

Requests for testing may be made for babies who are to be fostered or adopted. The birth mother should be informed and give her consent if this is to be performed. Where this consent is withheld, the person in loco parentis should do so. All neonatal screening prior to adoption has ethical implications. Why should adoptive parents be privy to information to which birth parents do not usually have access? In the case of HIV, they will also have information about the child's parent. Yet it could be argued that adoptive parents should have all the information necessary to enable them to care appropriately for their child? A child with HIV has a life-threatening condition, they will have to cope with the loss of that child, and raising a child with HIV has many challenges. It is still a socially unacceptable disease, and as such, parents have to cope with the effects of disclosure of the diagnosis to schools, friends and so on. The reaction they receive may be hostile and distressing. Problems of confidentiality may increase as the child becomes older and aware of his diagnosis, but not the effect it will have on others. Most adoption agencies do request HIV testing in order to place the child with an appropriate family who are open to caring for such a child.

Life expectancy and clinical management

Once the baby's seropositive status is known, the parents will want to know what the outcome is likely to be. It is the experience of many paediatricians that the outlook is poor for a proportion of babies. Paediatric AIDS has a shorter course than adult AIDS, with some babies dying in the first year of life. The Centers for Disease Control issued a separate classification for the signs of infection in perinatally acquired HIV infection. It was noted by Tovo *et al* (1992) that:

> the usefulness of this system, the reliability of the definition of AIDS in childhood, the frequency and prognostic importance of each disease pattern, and the probability of survival of perinatally infected children are not yet clearly established.

Using the Italian Register for HIV infection in children, consisting of 1887 children born to seropositive mothers they set out to analyse disease patterns and prognostic indicators. It appeared that of the seropositive children, 81.8 per cent had some clinical signs at the age of five months. However, these signs appeared significantly earlier in the children who died (a median of three months) than those who survived for a longer period (a median of six months). Almost 50 per cent of the infected children remained alive at nine years, and the median survival time was eight years. The researchers discovered three patterns of disease.

Table 8.2: Patterns of disease in paediatric AIDS
(Source: Tovo et al, 1992)

Hepatomegaly, splenomegaly, lymphadenopathy, parotitis, skin diseases, recurrent respiratory tract infections	mildest disease pattern
Lymphoid interstitial pneumonitis pattern	intermediate disease
Severe bacterial infections, progressive neurological disease, anaemia fever growth failure persistent oral candidiasis hepatitis cardiopathy	negative predictors of survival and associated with shorter survival time

It appears that there are two main forms that the disease takes: a shorter and more virulent form, leading to death within the first year, or a slower, less severe form with a much longer life expectancy. De Martino (1994) in a follow-up study using the Italian Register for HIV infection in children noted that long-term survival was associated with a moderate annual CD4 T-cell count drop, rather than an acute fall. However, long-term survivors did experience severe disease, but it did not inhibit their survival. The paper discusses the reasons why there may be two disease patterns. A genetically-determined immune response to HIV, similar to the milder form of the disease noted in adults is possible. Other factors which may have an impact are the mother's viral load and her immune status during pregnancy, method of feeding, and the timing of the mother-to-child transmission. It is thought that children who are infected early in pregnancy may have an accelerated and severe disease progression. The long-term survivors had higher birth weight, later onset of symptoms, and high CD8 counts suggesting that infection was acquired close to delivery.

A significant number of children with HIV suffer from neuro-developmental problems. Early studies in the USA gave figures as high as 90 per cent, and later European studies as 20 per cent (Alvarez *et al*, 1993). The authors report learning disabilities in six per cent of children, with 36 per cent having a significant language problem. It is highly probable that other factors are as important as HIV infection. Drug-use problems and other social and psychological factors form a major contribution.

The most common indicator disease of AIDS in children infected with HIV is Pneumocystis Carinii Pneumonia (PCP) (Ades *et al*, 1993; Hughes, 1991). PCP may also be the presenting clinical sign which leads to the initial diagnosis of HIV infection.

The Centers for Disease Control and Prevention issued guidelines for prophylaxis against Pneumocystis Carinii Pneumonia in children in 1991. The guidelines are based on estimation of CD4 T-cell count, which is age-related. The guidelines were based upon retrospective data collected from children following diagnosis. In adults, the CD4 T-cell count is a reliable indicator of risk for Pneumocystis Carinii Pneumonia. The European Collaborative Study Group sought to ex-amine if the CD4 T-cell count is as reliable in children using prospec-tive data collected from all children born to HIV infected mothers. They discovered that some children developed Pneumocystis Carinii Pneumonia when their CD4 T-cell count was higher than the thresh-old for prophylaxis, whereas 62 per cent of infected children who did not develop Pneumocystis Carinii Pneumonia had CD4 T-cell counts less than the level indicated for prophylaxis. Likewise, ten per cent of uninfected children also had lowered CD4 T-cell counts before the disappearance of the maternal antibody. Thus monitor-ing the CD4 T-cell count is of limited value in deciding when to commence prophylaxis. The authors suggest that prophylaxis is commenced in infants under six months of age as soon as HIV infec-tion is diagnosed. (Dunn, Newell *et al*, 1994) Prophylaxis may consist of trimethoprim-sulphamethoxazole (co-trimoxazole) or aero-solized pentamidine.

There is still no clear indication when to start anti-retroviral therapy in children. Zidovudine (AZT) may have benefits in the short-term, in reducing the incidence of opportunistic infection, but fails to se-cure a long-term effect (Vallee *et al*, 1993). An American study found that survival of children after routine use of AZT was no better than for those not treated, and that "early mortality has not decreased with advances in medical care" (Forsyth *et al*, 1993).

Breastfeeding

In 1985, a case-study reported HIV infection in a breastfed child whose mother had acquired infection postnatally via a blood transfu-sion (Ziegler et al, 1985). HIV had been isolated from breast-milk, but this report indicated that breastfeeding itself could be a route of transmission of infection. On top of the risks of transmission antenatally and perinatally, this added risk to the baby suggested that HIV positive mothers should not breastfeed.

This is not a simple recommendation, as many mothers do not know that they carry the virus. Bottlefeeding is not a panacea, it carries risks in itself, especially to infants born in settings where gastrointestinal infections are prevalent. In addition breast-milk has many factors protective to HIV and other infections.

The evidence of HIV transmission by breastfeeding raised questions about timing of maternal infection, timing of transmission, and the mechanism of transmission.

Analysis of studies in Lusaka, Rwanda, Zaire, and Australia demonstrated a risk of transmission of 29 per cent to their infants from mothers infected in the postnatal period (Dunn *et al*, 1992). It is understood that when an individual becomes infected there is a period of viraemia (Daar *et al*, 1988). The viral load within the breastmilk is likely to be greater at this time. In addition if the mother acquires the infection from a blood transfusion there is more likely to be a "more abrupt and severe viraemia". This is also when the baby's intestinal tract and immune system are immature (Lederman, 1992).

The mechanism of infection by breastfeeding is not well understood. It is not yet known whether infection occurs through cell-free virus in breast-milk or through cells infected by the virus. If the latter is true then colostrum, which is richer in macrophages than mature milk, may seem to be more infectious. Intervention studies where colostrum and early milk is expressed and discarded, and the baby given mature milk, are being considered to establish if this would reduce or prevent transmission. If the mechanism of transmission were more clearly known, it may become possible to offer advice to women on an individual basis about the risk of transmission.

There are several factors, however, which are known to increase the risk of transmission:
- presence of clinical AIDS;
- low CD4 count at delivery;
- PCR-positive cells in early milk;
- absent HIV-specific IgM;
- cracked nipples;
- breast abscess;
- damage to infant's mucosal surface.

The understanding that maternal infection acquired postnatally has such a high risk of transmission to the infant means that in areas of high prevalence of infection, women who are seronegative in pregnancy need to be counselled carefully about the risks of breastfeeding and transmission. However, the areas of highest prevalence are also those where bottlefeeding is the least safe.

The World Health Organisation (WHO) and UNICEF issued a consensus statement in 1992 giving recommendations on breastfeeding and HIV. It recognized that in settings where the primary cause of infant death is infectious diseases and malnutrition, breastfeeding should remain the standard advice, even when the risk of HIV infection is known. This is because the risk of mortality from other causes associated with non-breastfeeding is higher than the risk of the baby becoming infected through breast-milk. In settings where there is a safe alternative to breastfeeding, those women who are known to be infected with HIV should be advised not to breastfeed. The WHO also recommends that in these settings voluntary and confidential HIV testing should be made available to all women so that they can make informed choices about method of feeding.

Dunn and Newell (1992) in their review of studies of transmission by breastfeeding in mothers with known infection, described a risk of 14 per cent over and above the risk of transmission in pregnancy and at delivery. The Centres for Disease Control and Prevention in the USA recommended in 1985 that women with HIV infection should be advised not to breastfeed their babies. This advice, aimed at the American population, became accepted throughout the world, and other governments have endorsed the advice. However, breastfeeding may afford some protection to the infant from HIV infection, as it does from other viral diseases. It is understood that breast-milk contains IgA specific to HIV which protects the infant's mucosal surface by acting like an antiseptic paint. Breast-milk also contains an anti-CD4 binding factor which may afford the infant protection from infection (Van de Perre, 1993). In addition, children who are already infected may be protected, by the acquisition of passive antibodies, from other diseases which are a problem to immune-compromised infants. Breast-milk is known to give protection from diarrhoeal and respiratory tract infections, from other infections such as meningitis, and from allergies.

Lederman (1992) conducted a mathematical exercise to develop a quantitative assessment of the respective risks of breast and bottlefeeding and the overall effect on infant mortality. Taking the following factors into consideration:

- numbers of HIV infected mothers;
- rate of transmission;
- breastfeeding rate;
- rate of transmission by breastfeeding;
- infant mortality in HIV infected children;
- infant mortality in non-infected breastfed children;
- infant mortality in non-infected bottlefed children.

She concluded that,

> ...the failure to support breastfeeding could have a bigger impact on breastfeeding rates among much larger number of non-infected women than on the small number of infected women, many more of whom are unlikely to breastfeed whatever we advise. However, even if we were so successful at promoting breastfeeding that *all* women breastfed, even all infected women, mortality could very well be less than if all women bottlefed.

The identification of breastfeeding as a route of perinatal transmission has led to calls for antenatal testing so that women may be given the information and thus choice in their method of feeding (Dunn and Newell, 1992). A study in England demonstrated that 80 per cent of HIV positive women were undiagnosed at time of delivery (Ades *et al*, 1991). The criteria for routinely offering antenatal testing, however, should remain the same: it is appropriate and cost-effective in areas of high prevalence.

Current knowledge produces two opposing risks to infants, the risk of transmission of HIV from breastfeeding, and the risk of mortality incurred from non-breastfeeding causes. A balance is required between the prevention of transmission and the protection of the infant, afforded by breastfeeding. Studies would seem to advocate the promotion of breastfeeding generally within the population, but alternative feeding methods for infants of individuals with HIV infection, in settings where this is appropriate. In high prevalence areas, where the protection that breastfeeding affords is also necessary, studies are required into safe alternatives such as wet nursing, use of milk banks, pasteurisation, and cup feeding. In areas where the use of formula milk is a safe alternative, this is currently the appropriate advice.

Psychosocial aspects

Babies born into families with HIV infection may or may not be infected, but they will all be touched by the effects of the infection. Some babies may be born with clinical symptoms, or may develop them soon after birth. This may mean that they are hospitalized and separated from their mothers. If the baby is born to a drug-using mother, he or she will also require special care relating to this. Any separation of mother and baby in the postnatal period can interrupt or harm the bonding and attachment process.

Despite advances in neonatal testing, babies born to HIV positive mothers face an uncertain future. It may be many months before the diagnosis is confirmed or eliminated. This uncertainty may result in delayed acceptance of the baby.

If the mother is ill herself this brings additional difficulties to the development of the relationship. As well as coping with the uncertainty surrounding her child's future, she has to deal with her own personal issues. Sherr lists the obstacles which may hinder her ability to plan for the future care for her child: guilt, fear, anxiety, bereavement, lethargy, limited energy, lack of support and secrecy (Sherr, 1991).

Many babies and children born to HIV-infected mothers will require some form of care, foster or respite, increasing the possibility of emotional detachment. The lack of facilities for family care in hospitals increases the need for separations when in-patient treatment is required for the mother. The Mildmay Unit in London has built a special family unit, where a mother can be admitted accompanied by her children.

The physical condition of the parents, and the lifestyle sometimes surrounding drug-using women, may result in the infant having less physical and mental stimulation than other babies. Care for the family should take this into consideration, and provision for this be made.

Conclusion

The advance of the HIV disease appears to be relentless. The scientists work unstintingly, following their leads. Resources are poured into the work, (and money is certainly made in some quarters from the pandemic), but little concrete progress appears to be made. The numbers infected are still increasing and people continue to die. This is not to say that there has been no progress. Much has been achieved in the first decade of the disease. The organism responsible has been identified. We know how it acts and how it is transmitted. We know that between two out of three and four out of five babies will not become infected perinatally. We know that their mothers' condition will not necessarily deteriorate. We know that the outcomes and risks vary according to where you live.

But like every other virus, we do not have a cure. We do not even have an effective treatment. We do not yet have a vaccine. We do not have answers to many questions. So the future must lie not only in the search for a vaccine, for effective treatments and for effective measures to reduce and prevent transmission, but also in the prevention of the spread of this disease.

This is not a medical solution, but a political and social necessity. It involves a global acknowledgement that the problem exists, how it is spread, and how it is caused. This disease may have a biological cause, but the spread is of a largely social and political origin. Deprivation and poverty are inextricably linked with the spread, and will continue to be. Inequalities in health and wealth will foster the spread by causing inaccessibility to inadequately resourced health care, by ignorance and by social divisions.

The weapons against HIV and AIDS cannot rely solely on a would-be vaccine, and ineffective, vastly expensive drugs. They must include the armament of prevention: information; education; improved health; treatment of sexually transmitted diseases; and access to health care. Most importantly, they must include a cultural revolution, to acknowledge the position of women in the cycle of transmission, to acknowledge their responsibility for future generations by acknowledging their equal status in society. Only by empowering women to protect themselves can heterosexual spread be limited.

Young people, bearing the brunt of new infection, must also be involved in strategies for prevention. Gender and age-specific measures can be taken to increase their access to health care, to family planning and sexual health services. Youth is a time when danger represents excitement, and life is to be explored. Educational programmes should note this, as should the media, who could also take more responsibility for the power they hold by developing positive educational measures.

Lessons are continually being learnt and knowledge updated. Without a partnership of science and society, the size and the complexity of the problem will increase. It is vitally important not only to learn from pooled medical knowledge, but also from the hard facts of global inequalities, and the profound effect they have on us all.

References

Chapter 1

Dunn, D., Newell, M-L., Ades, A. and Peckham, C. (1992). 'Risk of human immunodeficiency virus type 1 transmission through breastfeeding', *Lancet,* Vol. 340, pp.585-88.

Padian, N., Shiboski, S. and Jewell, N. (1990). VI International Conference on AIDS, Abstracts, Vol 1, p.159.

Pratt, R. (1991). *AIDS: A Strategy for Nursing Care.* 3rd Edition. London: Edward Arnold.

Redfield, R. and Burke, D. (1988). 'HIV infection: the clinical picture'. In: *The Science of AIDS.* Readings from Scientific American. New York: W H Freeman.

Van de Perre, P. (1993). 'Postnatal transmission of HIV by breastfeeding', 2nd International Conference on HIV in Children and Mothers, Edinburgh, Abstracts, p.293.

Chapter 2

Chin, J. (1990). 'Current and future dimensions of the HIV/AIDS pandemic in women and children', *Lancet,* Vol. 336, pp.221-24

Merson, M. (1993). 'Women and children with HIV: the global experience (WHO)', 2nd International Conference on HIV in Children and Mothers, Edinburgh.

Chapter 3

CDC 1992.(1993). 'Revised clasification system for HIV infection and expanded surveillance case definition for AIDS among adolescents and adults', *MMWR,* Vol. 42, No. RR-17.

Chaisson, R., Stanton, D. *et al* (1993). 'Impact of the 1993 revision of the AIDS case definition on the prevalence of AIDS in a clinical setting', *AIDS,* Vol. 7, pp.857-62.

Chin, J. (1990). 'Current and future dimensions of the HIV/AIDS pandemic in women and children', *Lancet,* Vol. 336, pp.221-24

Lassoued, K., Clauvel, J-P. *et al* (1991). 'AIDS-associated Kaposi's Sarcoma in female patients', *AIDS,* Vol. 5, pp.877-80.

Rutherford, G.W., Lifson, A.R. *et al* (1990). 'Course of HIV-1 infection in a cohort of homosexual and bisexual men: an 11-year follow-up study', *BMJ,* Vol. 301, pp.1183-88.

Chapter 4

Boucher, C. (1993). 'Summary of WHO intervention workshop - chemotherapy. In: Peckham, C. and Newell, M-L. (Eds). *Measures to Decrease the Risk of Mother-to-Child Transmission of HIV Infection*. Reading: Colwood House Medical Publications.

Concorde Study (1994). 'Concorde: MRC/ANRS randomised double-blind controlled trial of immediate and deferred Zydovudine in symptom free HIV infection', *Lancet*, Vol. 343, No. 8902, pp. 871-77.

Dabis, F. (1993). 'Ghent - Mother to child transmission of HIV', 2nd International Conference on HIV in Children and Mothers, Edinburgh.

Dabis, F., Msellati, P. *et al* (1993). 'Estimating the rate of mother-to-child transmission of HIV. Report of a workshop on methodological issues - Ghent (Belgium)', *AIDS*, Vol. 7, pp.1139-48.

Goedert, J. *et al* (1991). 'The international registry of twins1991. International register of HIV-exposed twins: high risk of HIV-1 infection for the first born twins', *Lancet*, Vol. 338, pp.1471-75.

Hague, R., Mok, J. *et al* (1993). 'Maternal factors in HIV transmission', *International Journal of Sexually Transmitted Disease and AIDS*, Vol. 4, pp.142-46.

Hankins, C., Lapointe, N. *et al* (1993). 'Previous miscarriage/ therapeutic abortion associated with increased risk of mother-to-child HIV transmission', 2nd International Conference on HIV in Children and Mothers, Edinburgh, Poster/Abstracts, p.313.

Johnstone, F., MacCallum, L. *et al* (1988). 'Does infection with HIV affect the outcome of pregnancy?', *British Medical Journal*, Vol. 296, pp.467.

Lange, J. (1993). 'WHO and intervention studies'. In: Peckham, C. and Newell, M-L. (Eds). *Measures to Decrease the Risk of Mother-to-Child Transmission of HIV Infection*. Reading: Colwood House Medical Publications.

Lefevre, V., Lepage, E. and Ravina, J. H. (1993). 'Obstetrical risk facEuropean Collaborative Study (1992). 'Risk factors for mother-to-child transmission of HIV-1', *Lancet*, Vol. 339, pp.1007-12.

MacCallum, L., France, A., Jones, M. *et al* (1988). 'The effect of pregnancy on the progression of HIV infection', IVth International Conference on AIDS, Stockholm.

Mandelbrot, L. (1993). 'Lavage of birth canal'. In: Peckham, C. and Newell, M-L. (Eds). *Measures to Decrease the Risk of Mother-to-Child Transmission of HIV Infection*. Reading: Colwood House Medical Publications.

Mandelbrot, L., Cremieux, G. *et al* (1993). 'What determines seropositive women's choice to terminate or continue pregnancy?', 2nd International Conference on HIV in Children and Mothers, Edinburgh, Abstracts, p.301.

Mercey, D., Bewley, S. and Brocklehurst, P. (1993). *A Guide to HIV Infection and Childbearing*. Horsham: Avert.

Minkoff, H. L. (1987). 'Care of pregnant women with human immunodeficiency virus', *Journal of the American Medical Association,* Vol. 258, pp.2714-17.

Newell, M-L. (1993). 'European colaborative study - Risk factors for vertical transmission'. In: Peckham, C. and Newell, M-L. (Eds). *Measures to Decrease the Risk of Mother-to-Child Transmission of HIV Infection.* Reading: Colwood House Medical Publications.

Rossi, P. (1993). 'The role of hyperimmune-immunoglobulin'. In: Peckham, C. and Newell, M-L. (Eds). *Measures to Decrease the Risk of Mother-to-Child Transmission of HIV Infection.* Reading: Colwood House Medical Publications.

Schoenbaum, E., Davenny, K. and Selwyn, P. (1988). 'The impact of pregnancy on HIV-related disease'. In: Hudson, C.M. and Sharp, S. (Eds). *AIDS and Obstetrics & Gynaecology.* London: RCOG.

Sperling, R., Stratton, R., O'Sullivan, M. *et al* (1992). 'A survey of Zidovudine use in pregnant women with human immunodeficiency virus infection', *New England Journal of Medicine,* Vol. 326, pp.857-61.

Temmerman, M. (1993). 'HIV and pregnancy: double trouble!' 2nd International Conference on HIV in Children and Mothers, Edinburgh, Abstracts, p.292.

Temmerman, M., Chomba, E., *et al* (1994). 'Maternal human immunodeficiency virus-1 infection and pregnancy outcome', *Obstetric Gynecology,* Vol. 83, No. 4, pp.495-501.

Villari, P., Spirio, C., Chalmers, T.C., Lau, J., Sacks, S. (1993). 'Cesarean section to reduce perinatal transmission of human immunodeficiency virus: a meta-analysis.' *Outline Journal of Current Clinical Trails,* Vol. 2, July, Doc. No. 74.

Wahren, B. (1993). 'HIV vaccines'. In: Peckham, C. and Newell, M-L. (Eds). *Measures to Decrease the Risk of Mother-to-Child Transmission of HIV Infection.* Reading: Colwood House Medical Publications.

Zamora, L., Buira, E., Lonca, M. *et al* (1993). 'Influence of pregnancy in HIV infection', 2nd International Conference on HIV in Children and Mothers, Edinburgh, Poster/Abstracts, p.312.

Chapter 5

Concorde Study (1994). 'Concorde: MRC/ANRS randomised double-blind controlled trial of immediate and deferred Zydovudine in symptom free HIV infection', *Lancet,* Vol. 343, No. 8902, pp. 871-77.

Curtis, H. (1993). 'Who to test?', Pre-conference Symposium, 2nd International Conference on HIV in Children and Mothers, Edinburgh.

Department of Health (1992). 'Department of Health Guidance: Additional sites for HIV antibody testing; offering voluntary named HIV antibody testing to women receiving antenatal care, London.

Sherr, L. (1991). *HIV and AIDS in Mothers and Babies. A guide to Counselling.* London: Blackwell Scientific Publications.

Sunderland, A., Moroso, G., *et al* (1988). 'Influence of HIV infection on pregnancy decisions', IVth International Conference on AIDS, Stockholm.

UKCC (1992). *Code of Professional Conduct for the Nurse, Midwife and Health Visitor,* 3rd Edition, London:UKCC.

Chapter 6

Department of Health (1994). *AIDS - HIV infected Health Care Workers, Guid-*

ance on the Management of Infected Health Care Workers. Recommendations of the Expert Advisory Group on AIDS. London:DOH.

PHLS AIDS Centre (1993). 'Surveillance of occupational exposure: Information for health care workers and carers', Communicable Diseases Surveillance Centre, London, October.

Smith, J. and Grant, J. (1990). 'The incidence of glove puncture during caesarean section', *Journal of Obstetrics and Gynaecology,* Vol. 10, pp.317-18.

Chapter 7

Barlow, J. (1992). 'Social issues: an overview'. In: Bury, J.K., Morrison, V. and McLachlan, S. (Eds). *Working With Women and AIDS.* London: Tavistock/ Routledge.

Bisset, K. and Gray, J. (1992). 'Feelings and needs of women who are HIV positive'. In: Bury, J.K., Morrison, V. and McLachlan, S. (Eds). *Working With Women and AIDS.* London: Routledge.

Brierley, J. (1993). 'HIV and AIDS in Childbirth', *Mid Chron* Vol. 106, No. 1268, pp.317-25.

Briggs, G., Bodendorfer, T. *et al* (1983). *Drugs in Pregnancy and Lactation.* London: Williams and Wilkins.

Bury, J. K. (1989). 'Counselling women with HIV infection about pregnancy, heterosexual transmission and contraception', *British Journal of Family Planning,* Vol. 14, No. 4, pp. 116-22.

Cleary, J. and Young, A. (1993). 'The needs of women affected by HIV and AIDS', 2nd International Conference on HIV in Children and Mothers, Edinburgh, Abstracts, p.301.

Dick, S. (1992). 'Positive support', *Nursing Times,* Vol. 88, No. 44, pp. 46-48.

Johnson, A. M. (1988). 'Heterosexual transmission of human immunodeficiency virus', *British Medical Journal,* Vol. 296, pp.1017-20.

Johnstone, F. D. (1992). 'Management of pregnancy in women with HIV infection', *British Journal of Hospital Medicine,* Vol. 48, No. 10, pp.664-70.

Mercey, D., Bewley, S. and Brocklehurst, P. (1993). *A Guide to HIV Infection and Childbearing.* Horsham: Avert.

Thomson, K. (1992). 'Being positive'. In: Bury, J.K., Morrison, V. and McLachlan, S. (Eds). *Working With Women and AIDS.* London: Tavistock/ Routledge.

World Health Organisation (1987). 'Report of a meeting on contraceptive methods and HIV infection', *Special Programme of Research, Development and Research Training in Human Reproduction and Special Programme on AIDS,*Geneva.

Chapter 8

Ades, A., Davison, C., *et al* (1993). 'Vertically transmitted HIV infection in the British Isles, *British Medical Journal,* Vol. 306, pp.1296-99.Alvarez, M., Papola, P. and Cohen, H. (1993). Neurodevelopmental abnormalities in school-age children with HIV infection', 2nd International Conf. on HIV in Children and Mothers, Edinburgh, Abstracts, p.308.

Bredberg-Raden, U., Urassa, E., *et al* (1993). 'Early diagnosis of HIV-1 infection in infants in tanzania', 2nd International Conference on HIV in Children and Mothers, Edinburgh, Abstracts, p.305.

Caselli, D., Marconi, M. *et al* (1993). 'HIV specific IgG3 for early diagnosis in children born to HIV-infected mothers', 2nd International Conference on HIV in Children and Mothers, Edinburgh, Abstracts, p. 305.

Daar, E., Moudgil, T., *et al* (1988). 'Transient high levels of viraemia in patients with primary human immunodeficiency virus type 1 infection', *New England Journal of Medicine*, Vol. 324, pp.961-64.

De Martino, M. and the Italian Register for HIV Infection in Children (1994). 'Features of children perinatally infected with HIV-1 surviving longer than 5 years', *Lancet*, Vol. 343, pp.191-95.

Dunn, D., Newell, M-L., *et al* (1992). 'Risk of human immunodeficiency virus type 1 transmission through breast feeding', *Lancet*, Vol. 340, pp. 585-88.

European Collaborative Study, Dunn, D., Newell, M-L. *et al* (1994). 'CD4 T cell count as predictor of *pneumocystis carinii* pneumonia in children born to mothers infected with HIV', *British Medical Journal*, Vol. 308, pp.437-40.

Forsyth, B., O'Connor, T. *et al* (1993). 'Survival of HIV-infected children', 2nd International Conference on HIV in Children and Mothers, Edinburgh, Abstracts, p.306.

Garburg-Chenon, A., Segondy, M. *et al* (1993). 'Virus isolation, polymerase chain reaction and *in vitro* antibody production for the diagnosis of paediatric human immunodeficiency virus infection', *Journal of Virological Methods*, Vol. 42, No. 1, pp.117-25.

Hughes, W. T. (1991). 'Pneumocystis carinii pneumonia: new approaches to diagnosis, treatment, and prevention', *Pediatric Infectious Disease Journal*, Vol. 10, pp.391-99.

Lederman, S. A. (1992). 'Estimating infant mortality from human immunodeficiency virus and other causes in breast-feeding and bottle-feeding populations', *Pediatrics*, Vol. 89, No. 2, pp.290-96.

Perez-Alvarez, L., Gurbindo-Gutierrez, D. *et al* (1992). 'Early diagnosis of HIV infection in children born to seropositive mothers'(Abstract). *An. Esp. Pediatr.*, Vol. 37, No. 3, pp.223-27.

Sherr, L. (1991). *HIV and AIDS in Mothers and Babies. A guide to Counselling*. London:Blackwell Scientific Publications.

Tovo, P., De Martino, M., *et al* (1992). Prognostic factors and survival in children with perinatal HIV-1 infection, and the Italian register for HIV infection in children', *Lancet*, Vol. 339, pp.1249-53.

Vallee, D. (1993). 'Early treatment by Azidothymine in perinatally HIV infected children', 2nd International Conference on HIV in Children and Mothers, Edinburgh, Abstracts, p.326.

World Health Organisation (1992). 'Consensus statement from the WHO/UNICEF consultation on HIV transmission and breast-feeding', WHO/GPA/92.1.

Ziegler, J., Cooper, D. *et al* (1985). 'Postnatal transmission of AIDS-associated retrovirus from mother to infant', *Lancet*, Vol. II, pp.896-98.

Appendix I

Conditions included in the 1993 AIDS Surveillance Case Definition

- Candidiasis of bronchi, trachea, or lungs
- Candidiasis, esophageal
- Cervical cancer, invasive[1]
- Coccidioidomycosis, disseminated or extrapulmonary
- Cryptococcosis, extrapulmonary
- Cryptosporidiosis, chronic intestinal (> one month's duration)
- Cytomegalovirus disease (other than liver, spleen or nodes)
- Cytomegalovirus retinitis (with loss of vision)
- Encephalopathy, HIV-related
- Herpes simplex: chronic ulcer(s) (> one month's duration); or bronchitis, pneumonitis, or esophagitis
- Histoplasmosis, disseminated or extrapulmonary
- Isosporiasis, chronic intestinal (> one month's duration)
- Kaposi's Sarcoma
- Lymphoma, Burkitt's (or equivalent term)
- Lymphoma, immunoblastic (or equivalent term)
- Lymphoma, primary, of brain
- *Mycobacterium avium* complex or *M. kansasii*, disseminated or extrapulmonary
- *Mycobacterium tuberculosis*, any site (pulmonary[1] or extrapulmonary)
- *Mycobacterium*, other species or unidentified species, disseminated or extrapulmonary
- *Pneumocystis carinii* pneumonia
- Pneumonia, recurrent[1]
- Progressive multifocal leukoencephalopathy
- *Salmonella* septicemia, recurrent
- Toxoplasmosis of brain
- Wasting syndrome due to HIV

[1]Added in the 1993 expansion of the AIDS surveillance case definition.

Appendix II

AIDS/HIV INFECTED HEALTH CARE WORKERS: GUIDANCE ON THE MANAGEMENT OF INFECTED HEALTH CARE WORKERS

Key Recommendations

1. All health care workers should routinely follow general infection control guidelines and adopt safer working practices to prevent transmission of HIV infection. (Paragraph 3.1)

2. Health care workers have an ethical duty to protect patients. Those who believe they may have been exposed to infection with HIV in their personal life or during the course of their work must seek medical advice and if appropriate, diagnostic HIV antibody testing. (Paragraph 4.2)

3. HIV infected health care workers should not undertake procedures that may place patients at even a remote risk of infection. These are defined in this guidance as exposure prone invasive procedures. (Paragraph 3.6)

4. Health care workers found to be infected must seek appropriate medical and occupational advice and those who perform or assist in exposure prone invasive procedures must obtain further advice on their work practices which may need to be modified or restricted to protect their patients. (Paragraph 4.2 and 6.1)

5. HIV infected health care workers who continue to work with patients must remain under close medical supervision and receive appropriate medical and occupational advice as their circumstances change. (Paragraph 4.3)

6. Workers who are found to be HIV positive and who have performed exposure prone invasive procedures whilst infected must cease these activities immediately and inform their employing or contracting authority so that they can decide what, if any, action is necessary. (Paragraph 4.5 and 4.6)

7.   Physicians who are aware that infected health care workers under their care have not sought or followed advice to modify their practice, must inform the employing authority and appropriate regulatory body. Where a health care worker is not a member of one of these bodies the physician will inform only the employing authority. (Paragraph 4.7)

8.   Health Authorities and NHS Trusts must bring to the attention of current and new employees including Agency staff and independent contractors the professional regulatory bodies notices of ethical responsibilities and occupational guidance for HIV infected health care workers, and must ensure, as must medical colleges and universities, that students in training are appraised of the relevant professional statements. (Paragraph 5.1)

9.   The Expert Advisory Group on AIDS [EAGA] and the UK Advisory Panel on HIV infected health care workers recommend that all patients who have undergone an exposure prone invasive procedure where the infected health care worker was the sole or main operator should, as far as is practicable, be notified of this. (Paragraph 8.1)

10.   All matters arising from and relating to the employment of HIV infected health care workers should be coordinated through a consultant in occupational health medicine. (Paragraph 6.2)

11.   Employers must make every effort to arrange suitable alternative work and retraining, or where appropriate, early retirement, for HIV infected health care workers. (Paragraph 5.4)

12.   Employers have a duty to keep information on the health, including HIV status, of employees confidential and are not legally entitled to disclose an employee has HIV infection except where the employee consents, unless to do so would be in the public interest. Those making such a disclosure may be required to justify their decision. This duty does not end with the death of the worker. (Paragraph 5.2, 5.3, Section 10)

Index